CRANIAL NERVES
Functional Anatomy

Cranial nerves are involved in head and neck function, and processes such as eating, speech and facial expression. This clinically oriented survey of cranial nerve anatomy and function was written for students of medicine, dentistry and speech therapy, but will also be useful for postgraduate physicians and general practitioners, and specialists in head and neck healthcare (surgeons, dentists, speech therapists, etc.). After an introductory section surveying cranial nerve organization and tricky basics such as ganglia, nuclei and brain stem pathways, the nerves are considered in functional groups: (1) for chewing and facial sensation; (2) for pharynx and larynx, swallowing and phonation; (3) autonomic components, taste and smell; (4) vision and eye movements; and (5) hearing and balance. In each chapter, the main anatomical features of each nerve are followed by clinical aspects and details of clinical testing. Simple line diagrams accompany the text. Detailed anatomy is not given.

Stanley Monkhouse is Anatomist at the University of Nottingham at Derby (Graduate Entry Medicine). He has been an examiner at the Royal Colleges of Surgeons of England and Ireland; at the Universities of Nottingham, Leeds, Newcastle-upon-Tyne, London, Belfast, Dublin (Trinity College), National University of Ireland, King AbdulAziz University (Jeddah, Saudi Arabia), Amman (Jordan) and King Faisal University (Dammam, Saudi Arabia).

CRANIAL NERVES

Functional Anatomy

STANLEY MONKHOUSE

MA, MB, BChir, PhD

University of Nottingham Medical School at Derby

Sometime Professor of Anatomy at the Royal College of
Surgeons in Ireland; Lecturer in Human Morphology at the
University of Nottingham; and Clinical Assistant in Ear Nose
and Throat, Queen's Medical Centre, Nottingham

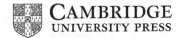

CAMBRIDGE
UNIVERSITY PRESS

CAMBRIDGE UNIVERSITY PRESS
Cambridge, New York, Melbourne, Madrid, Cape Town, Singapore,
São Paulo, Delhi

Cambridge University Press
The Edinburgh Building, Cambridge CB2 8RU, UK

Published in the United States of America by
Cambridge University Press, New York

www.cambridge.org
Information on this title: www.cambridge.org/9780521615372

First published 2006

A catalogue record for this publication is available from the British Library

ISBN 978-0-521-61537-2 paperback

Transferred to digital printing 2009

CONTENTS

FIGURES

TABLES

ACKNOWLEDGEMENTS

This book grew from notes first written in 1992 for medical and surgical students at the Royal College of Surgeons in Ireland. Comments from students over the years helped me to modify the text, and I am therefore greatly indebted to those whom I have taught. The notes were condensed for inclusion in my textbook Clinical Anatomy (first published by Churchill Livingstone, 2001), and I acknowledge with thanks the cooperation of staff at Elsevier in allowing the use of the original notes here.

There are several people who deserve my special thanks. The first is Eric Clarke who goaded me into action in 1992 and who has been a constant source of encouragement and practical help. The second is Dr Gordon Wright MA, MD, Fellow of Clare College, Cambridge, who in 1970–1971 taught me neuroanatomy with great wit and style, and who responded to my request for constructive criticism of an earlier version of the text. Of course, I bear sole responsibility for errors. I look forward to receiving constructive criticism from others. And finally, I thank Pauline Graham and her colleagues at Cambridge University Press.

I would like to think that this book would have met with the approval of Maxwell Marsden Bull MA, MD, sometime Fellow and Senior Tutor of Queens' College, Cambridge. He had a great gift for expository and analytical teaching, and he showed me that *educare* and *delectare* can be synonymous.

Stanley Monkhouse
Derby 2005

A NOTE TO THE READER

For those of you who will become physicians and general practitioners, cranial nerves are important. Undergraduate anatomy is probably the last time you will study their anatomy, so you need to get the hang of it first time round. This book was written with you in mind. It assumes that you will have some understanding of the functional anatomy of the spinal cord, spinal nerves, trunk and limbs.

If you want to jump straight to the main business of cranial nerves, skip Part I which deals with their organization. I advise you to try reading it sometime, though, because it covers topics that students find troublesome but which aid understanding if properly appreciated. If you persevere with Part I you might be rewarded with, at the very least, a warm inward glow when the light finally dawns on some previously murky corner.

Parts II–V deal with the functional anatomy of the nerves. Rather than work through them from first to twelfth, the book considers them according to function. You will encounter them much as would an ingested morsel of food. This is unorthodox: it does, though, lend spice and relevance.

There are several approaches to cranial nerves: the embryological and evolutionary, the analytical, and that which numbs the senses with topographical detail. Although a little of all these is desirable, none alone is adequate. The principal emphasis of this book is on clinically useful information, but because understanding is aided by some analysis and embryology, the book is more than just a list of points for cramming. I hope that the inclusion of some explanatory material will stimulate you whilst not obscuring the basics. It is by no means the last word on the subject, and I expect that research neuroanatomists will throw up their hands in horror at some of the generalizations it contains. It is unavoidable that some material appears more than once, but I hope that this repetition will reinforce rather than bore.

PART I

ORGANIZATION OF THE
CRANIAL NERVES

Chapter 1

GENERAL CONSIDERATIONS

1.1　Cranial nerves and their functions (Table 1.1)

Cranial nerves arise from the brain as twelve pairs. They pass through or into the cranial bones (thus *cranial* nerves) and are numbered I to XII roughly in order from top (rostral) to bottom (caudal). Their functions are those of the head: some are concerned with awareness of, and communication with, the environment; and some are concerned with sustenance, the gut tube and movements associated with it.

1.2　Cranial nerves and spinal nerves are differently constituted

Cranial nerves are not equivalent to spinal nerves. All spinal nerves have similar functions and carry similar types of nerve fibre (motor, sensory, autonomic, etc.). This is not so for cranial nerves:
- Some cranial nerves contain only sensory fibres, some contain only motor fibres, and some contain both.
- Some cranial nerves convey parasympathetic fibres, some convey taste fibres, some convey both, and some neither.

Cranial nerves exhibit great variety and functional specialization. This is evident in Table 1.1 which summarizes their numbers, names and main functions. Learn this table without further ado, and make sure that you can use names and numbers

Table 1.1. Synopsis of cranial nerves.

	Name	Type	Principal clinical function (other functions in parentheses)
I	Olfactory	Sensory	Smell
II	Optic	Sensory	Vision
III	Oculomotor	Motor	Movements of eyeball: most orbital muscles. See also IV, VI (parasympathetic: ciliary muscle, accommodation of lens, etc.; iris muscle, pupilloconstriction)
IV	Trochlear	Motor	Movements of eyeball: superior oblique muscle. See also III, VI
V	Trigeminal		
	Va: Ophthalmic	Sensory	Sensation from eyeball, anterior scalp, upper face
	Vb: Maxillary	Sensory	Sensation from nasal cavity and sinuses, palate, mid face, maxillary teeth
	Vc: Mandibular	Mixed	Muscles of mastication, tensor tympani Sensation from chin, temple, oral cavity, tongue, temporomandibular joint (TMJ), mandibular teeth, ear, proprioception from muscles of mastication
VI	Abducens	Motor	Movements of eyeball: lateral rectus muscle. See also III, IV

	Name	Type	Functions
VII	Facial	Mixed	Muscles of facial expression, stapedius (middle ear) (parasympathetic: lacrimal, nasal, palatine, submandibular, sublingual glands) (taste: anterior tongue)
VIII	Vestibulocochlear	Sensory	Hearing, balance
IX	Glossopharyngeal	Mixed	Sensation from oropharynx, posterior tongue, carotid body and sinus (taste: posterior tongue) (muscle: stylopharyngeus) (parasympathetic: parotid gland)
X	Vagus	Mixed	Muscles of larynx, pharynx (phonation, swallowing) Sensation from larynx, pharynx, hypopharynx, heart, lungs, abdominal viscera (taste: epiglottic region, hypopharynx) (parasympathetic: cardiac muscle; muscles and glands of foregut and midgut: intestinal activity)
XI	Accessory	Motor	Muscles: sternocleidomastoid, trapezius
XII	Hypoglossal	Motor	Tongue muscles and movements

interchangeably: in the clinical situation the nerves are often referred to by number only.

1.3   Olfactory and optic nerves are not "proper" nerves

The first two cranial nerves, olfactory and optic, are not really nerves at all: they are brain outgrowths, and so many general terms are not appropriate for them. They are considered separately in Chapters 18 and 20.

1.4   Attachments of cranial nerves (Table 1.2; Figs 1.1 and 1.2)

I and II are attached to the cerebral hemispheres, and III to XII to the brain stem (midbrain, pons and medulla). The three enlargements of the neural tube from which the brain develops are as follows:

Forebrain, further subdivided into two components:
telencephalon (the cerebral hemispheres) and diencephalon
(the thalamic structures surrounding the third ventricle).
Midbrain, or mesencephalon.
Hindbrain: pons, cerebellum and medulla.

Cranial nerves arising from the forebrain: I, II
The olfactory nerve (I) is attached to the under surface of the frontal lobe; its connections pass to the temporal lobe and elsewhere.

The optic nerve (II) is an outgrowth of the diencephalon and is attached to structures in the wall and floor of the third ventricle.

Cranial nerves arising from the midbrain: III, IV
The oculomotor nerve (III) arises from the interpeduncular fossa on the ventral aspect of the midbrain.

Table 1.2. Attachments and foramina of cranial nerves.

Brain attachment	Nerve	Foramen or canal (cranial bone in brackets)
Forebrain		
Telencephalon: limbic system	I	Cribriform plate (ethmoid)
Diencephalon: lateral geniculate body	II	Optic canal (sphenoid)
Midbrain		
Upper midbrain, ventral, interpeduncular fossa	III	Superior orbital fissure (sphenoid)
Lower midbrain, dorsal, below inferior colliculi	IV	Superior orbital fissure (sphenoid)
Hindbrain		
Pons, lateral aspect	V	Va: superior orbital fissure (sphenoid)
		Vb: foramen rotundum (sphenoid)
		Vc: foramen ovale (sphenoid)
Pontomedullary junction		
Near midline	VI	Superior orbital fissure (sphenoid)
Cerebellopontine angle	VII	Internal acoustic meatus, facial canal, stylomastoid foramen (temporal)
Cerebellopontine angle	VIII	Internal acoustic meatus (temporal)
Medulla		
Rootlets, lateral to inferior olive, extending down to cervical cord	IX, X, XI	Jugular foramen (between occipital and temporal bones)
Rootlets between pyramid and olive	XII	Hypoglossal canal (occipital)

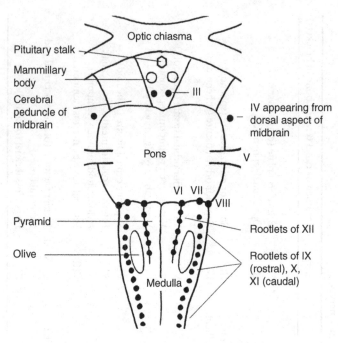

Fig. 1.1 Attachments of cranial nerves. Anterior view: study with
        brain stem specimen.

The trochlear nerve (IV) is the only cranial nerve to arise from
the dorsal aspect of the brain stem; it arises just below the inferior
colliculus.

Cranial nerves arising from the hindbrain: V–XII
The trigeminal nerve (V) arises from the lateral aspect of the
mid pons.

The abducens (VI), facial (VII) and vestibulocochlear (VIII)
nerves arise from the pontomedullary junction: VI is close to the
midline, VII and VIII arise laterally in the cerebellopontine angle.

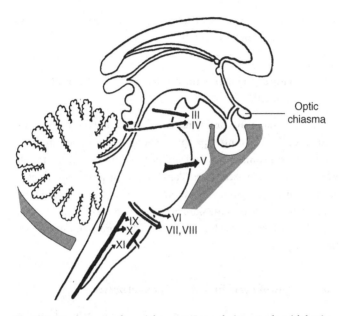

Fig. 1.2 Attachments of cranial nerves. Lateral view: study with brain
stem specimen.

The glossopharyngeal (IX), vagus (X) and accessory (XI) nerves
arise from the medulla by a longitudinal series of rootlets lateral to
the olive.

The hypoglossal (XII) nerve also arises from the medulla by a
longitudinal series of rootlets, but medial to the olive – between it
and the pyramid.

Medial–lateral relationships in brain stem attachments
Nerves which are attached close to the midline are exclusively motor:
III, IV, VI, XII (ignore for the moment the fact that IV emerges dor-
sally). Nerves emerging more laterally are either mixed – V, VII, IX,

X; or exclusively sensory – VIII. The significance of these relationships is explained in Section 1.10.

1.5   Central/peripheral: the border is NOT at the skull foramen!

Central means brain and spinal cord – the central nervous
system (CNS). The central/peripheral boundary is at the margin of
the brain and spinal cord, and not at the skull foramen through
which the nerve passes. Thus, components of peripheral nerves,
such as sensory ganglia and Schwann cells, may be found within the
cranial cavity or within the skull bones themselves on that part of a
cranial nerve between the brain and the skull foramen through which
the nerve passes.

1.6   Types of nerve fibre within cranial nerves

The simplest classification of fibre types is based on the
direction of impulse: motor (efferent) or sensory (afferent). Other
classifications are also helpful:
(a) The mode of control: voluntary or involuntary.
(b) The embryological origin of the structure innervated: somatic
     (somite, body wall) or visceral (gut tube, internal organs).
(c) The distribution in the body: general (widespread) or special
     (restricted to the head and neck).

Motor nerves: voluntary/involuntary
It is useful to classify motor nerves as voluntary or involuntary. Significant motor disorders result from the interruption of
pathways to voluntary muscles, and it is useful to know these
pathways.

Motor nerves: somatic/visceral

An embryological distinction is also useful: somatic motor, supplying body wall muscles mainly derived from somites, and visceral
motor, supplying muscle associated with yolk sac derivatives and
internal organs. Even though research casts doubt on the validity of
this distinction, it is helpful conceptually and it enables us to predict
with some accuracy the position of nerve roots and motor nuclei
within the brain stem (Sections 1.10 and 2.7).

**Sensory nerves: somatic/visceral is not a particularly useful
distinction**

Somatic sensation is sensation from body wall structures (soma:
body): in cranial nerves, it includes that from the skin and oral cavity (except taste). Visceral sensation includes that from the alimentary
canal (except the mouth) and taste. The somatic/visceral distinction is based not upon the nature of the peripheral nerve or neuron, but upon how the information is handled once inside the CNS:
brain stem connections of somatic sensation are different from
those of visceral sensation (Section 4.2).

1.7   Ganglion and nucleus: beware of confusion! (Fig. 1.3)

Ganglia and nuclei are easily confused. Both contain nerve
cell bodies, and some cranial nerves are associated with both a ganglion and a nucleus with the same name. For example, the trigeminal nerve (V) is associated with the trigeminal ganglion and several
trigeminal nuclei, and the vestibulocochlear nerve (VIII) is associated with vestibular and cochlear ganglia and vestibular and cochlear
nuclei. Furthermore, the term ganglion is applied to two different
structures associated with nerves. Explanation is necessary.

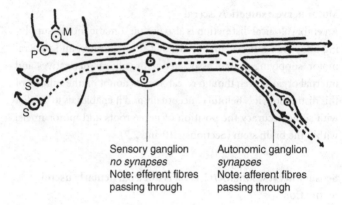

Sensory ganglion   Autonomic ganglion
no synapses   *synapses*
Note: efferent fibres   Note: afferent fibres
passing through   passing through

Fig. 1.3 Ganglia and nuclei.

In the central nuclei:

M: a group of cell bodies like this would form a motor
   nucleus, with cell bodies of lower motor neurons for
   voluntary motor activity.

P: a group of cell bodies like this would form a parasympathetic nucleus, with cell bodies of preganglionic parasympathetic neurons.

S: a group of cell bodies like these would form *either* a
   somatic sensory nucleus, for example trigeminal sensory
   nuclei for cutaneous sensation; *or* a visceral sensory
   nucleus, for example nucleus of solitary tract. In both cases
   the cell bodies of the primary sensory neurons would be in
   a peripheral sensory ganglion like that illustrated.

A ganglion is simply a swelling. Thus, in a nerve, ganglion means
a swelling on the nerve. It is used to mean the swelling caused by a
collection of nerve cell bodies on a peripheral nerve: cell bodies take
up more space than fibres, so a collection of cell bodies will cause a
swelling.

A nucleus is an aggregation of cell bodies in the CNS (exception: basal ganglia of the brain, the term being of historical significance; basal nuclei is better).

Ganglia are peripheral; nuclei are central.

1.8 Ganglia (Fig. 1.3)

A ganglion is a collection of nerve cell bodies associated with a peripheral nerve. There are two types of ganglia: those with synapses and those without.

1 *Ganglia with synapses: autonomic ganglia*

These are found on autonomic (visceral motor) pathways, and are thus autonomic ganglia. Autonomic neurons in cranial nerves are parasympathetic. Preganglionic neurons convey impulses from brain stem nuclei and synapse with postganglionic neurons, the cell bodies of which constitute the ganglia. (For sympathetic ganglia, see Chapter 19.)

2 *Ganglia without synapses: sensory ganglia*

Nearly all primary sensory neurons have their cell bodies in peripheral ganglia – sensory ganglia. Primary sensory neurons are usually pseudounipolar: that is to say, the single axon which arises from the cell body bifurcates into a peripheral process which passes towards the receptor, and a central process which passes towards the brain. There are no synapses in sensory ganglia. An example of this type of ganglion is found on every nerve containing sensory fibres; on spinal nerves they are dorsal root ganglia.

Note that each ganglion is either a sensory ganglion or an autonomic ganglion; there is no such thing as a mixed autonomic and sensory ganglion.

Table 1.3. Head and neck ganglia.

Sensory Cell bodies of primary sensory neurons (no synapses)	Autonomic (Motor) Cell bodies of postganglionic neurons (synapses)	
	Parasympathetic	Sympathetic

• Trigeminal V
• Geniculate VII
• Cochlear (spiral) VIII
• Vestibular VIII
• Superior and petrosal
  (inferior) of IX
• Jugular (superior) and
  nodose (inferior) of X
• Dorsal root ganglia of C 1–8
	• Ciliary
	• Pterygopalatine
	• Submandibular
	• Otic
		• Superior, middle
		and inferior
		cervical ganglia
		of sympathetic
		chain

Ganglia associated with cranial nerves (Table 1.3; Fig. 1.3)
Since some cranial nerves contain both sensory and parasympathetic fibres, they are associated with both sensory and parasympathetic ganglia:
• One cranial nerve is associated with only a parasympathetic ganglion: III contains fibres synapsing in the ciliary ganglion.
• One cranial nerve is associated with only sensory ganglia: VIII.
• Three cranial nerves are associated with both types of ganglion: V, VII, IX.
• The vagus nerve (X) is associated with both types of ganglia but its parasympathetic fibres synapse in autonomic ganglia of the thorax and abdomen, not in any parasympathetic ganglia of the head.
This is further complicated by the fact that although parasympathetic impulses leave the brain stem in III, VII, IX and X, those in

III, VII and IX are distributed to target organs in branches of V, to which their peripheral ganglia are attached. Don't worry about all these now – wait for Chapter 17!

1.9 Nuclei

A nucleus is a collection in the central grey matter of cell bodies of neurons serving similar functions. There are both motor and sensory nuclei.

1 *Motor nucleus: cell bodies of lower motor neurons*
Brain stem motor nuclei consist of cell bodies of motor neurons, the axons of which pass into a cranial nerve. Synapsing on these nuclei are motor neurons from higher brain centres.

2 *Sensory nucleus: cell bodies of secondary sensory neurons*
Brain stem sensory nuclei consist of cell bodies of secondary sensory neurons. The central processes of primary sensory neurons pass into the CNS to synapse in these sensory nuclei with the cell bodies of secondary sensory neurons. The axons of the secondary sensory neurons ascend to the contralateral thalamus and other higher centres.

1.10 Position of nuclei within the brain stem

In the developing neural tube, motor components are in the ventral portion (basal lamina) and sensory components in the dorsal portion (alar lamina). These are separated by the sulcus limitans on the wall of the central canal. Within both basal and alar laminae, visceral elements develop near the sulcus, and somatic elements towards the dorsal and ventral margins. Thus, from ventral to dorsal the components are found in the following order: somatic motor, visceral motor, visceral sensory and somatic sensory.

In the brain stem, this is preserved in a modified fashion. During development, it is as if the dorsal aspects of the brain stem were forcibly parted, each side being pushed laterally, by the enlarging central canal which becomes the fourth ventricle. The sequence somatic motor, visceral motor, visceral sensory, somatic sensory in the brain stem is therefore not so much ventral to dorsal as medial to lateral. Thus somatic motor nerves (e.g. III, XII) arise near the midline, nerves with visceral components (e.g. V, VII, IX, X) arise further laterally, and the entirely sensory VIII most lateral of all. Refer again to Section 1.4.

Chapter 2

CRANIAL NERVE MOTOR FIBRES AND NUCLEI

2.1   Motor fibres

Motor fibres are present in all cranial nerves except I, II and VIII.

2.2   Classification of motor components in cranial nerves

In spinal nerves, it is useful to distinguish between somatic and visceral motor fibres. This is based on the embryological origin of the muscle innervated.

Somatic motor (voluntary) fibres innervate muscles which develop from somites: striated muscle. Cell bodies are the ventral horn cells of the spinal cord grey matter. These muscles are under voluntary control.

Visceral motor (autonomic, involuntary) fibres innervate muscles which develop in association with the gut tube and its derivatives (e.g. bronchial tree), in glands, hair follicles and the heart. Except for cardiac muscle, it is smooth or non-striated. It is involuntary.

Thus, in the trunk and limbs voluntary may be loosely equated with striated and somatic, and involuntary with smooth and visceral.

2.3   Additional component in cranial nerves: for branchial arches

In the head and neck there is an additional group of muscles which are striated and are under voluntary control, but are classed

as visceral because they develop in association with the cranial end
of the gut tube. These are derivatives of the branchial or pharyngeal
arches. Branchial arch muscles are concerned only with the cephalic
end of the gut tube and have no equivalents below the neck; they are
innervated by branchiomotor fibres, found only in cranial nerves,
which originate from branchiomotor nuclei in the brain stem.

2.4   Types of motor nerve fibres

There are thus three types of motor nerve fibres in cranial
nerves:
1 Voluntary – somatic.
2 Voluntary – visceral – branchiomotor (special visceral; special
   because confined to the head and neck).
3 Involuntary – visceral – parasympathetic (general visceral; general
   because distributed more widely).
Remember: In cranial nerves visceral cannot be equated exclusively
with autonomic or involuntary.

Motor fibres supplying voluntary muscles are found in all cranial
nerves except I, II and VIII. Cranial nerve motor fibres are either
somatic or visceral (somatic and visceral fibres are never found in
the same nerve).

2.5   Motor fibres in cranial nerves

• Somatic motor: III, IV, VI, XII:
  – Extrinsic ocular muscles which move the eyeball and upper eye-
    lid: oculomotor (III), trochlear (IV) and abducens (VI) nerves.
  – Tongue muscles: hypoglossal nerve (XII).
• Branchiomotor: V, VII, IX, X (XI) (Table 2.1).

Table 2.1. Branchial arches, muscles and nerves.

Branchial arch	Muscles	Nerves
First	Muscles of mastication, etc.	Mandibular Vc
Second	Muscles of facial expression, etc.	Facial VII
Third	Stylopharyngeus	Glossopharyngeal IX
Fourth	Pharyngeal muscles	Pharyngeal branches of X
Sixth	Laryngeal muscles	Recurrent laryngeal of X

– The five branchial arches consist of ridges of mesoderm passing ventral–dorsal on either side of the foregut at the head end
  of the embryo. For reasons which need not concern us, these
  are numbered, cranial–caudal, as I, II, III, IV and VI. Each
  branchial arch gives rise to skeletal structures, muscles, nerves
  and arteries, the muscles of an arch being innervated by the
  nerve of that arch.

Axons and cell bodies of voluntary motor nerves

For both somatic and branchiomotor voluntary fibres, axons in
peripheral nerves pass without interruption from cell bodies in the
brain stem motor nuclei to the muscles of destination. These neurons are called lower motor neurons. Note that their cell bodies are
in the central nervous system.

2.6   Parasympathetic components of cranial nerves

Parasympathetic fibres emerge from the brain in only
four cranial nerves: III, VII, IX and X, and are delivered to their
destinations in branches of V. They innervate the ciliary and iris

muscles of the eyeball, and the salivary, lacrimal, nasal and palatal glands. They are arranged with two peripheral neurons: pre- and postganglionic. Cell bodies of preganglionic neurons are in brain stem parasympathetic nuclei, and their axons synapse on postganglionic neurons in peripheral parasympathetic ganglia. See Chapter 17.

2.7 Brain stem motor nuclei (Table 2.2; Fig. 2.1)

Axons of cranial nerve motor neurons originate from brain stem nuclei of three types corresponding to the embryological origin of the muscle groups:

1 *Somatic nuclei*: These are close to the midline, equivalent to spinal cord ventral horn cells. Somatic nuclei are oculomotor, trochlear, abducens and hypoglossal nuclei.

2 *Branchiomotor nuclei*: These develop lateral to somatic nuclei, between them and parasympathetic nuclei. Branchiomotor nuclei are trigeminal motor, facial motor and the nucleus ambiguus (and probably its cervical extension for the spinal accessory nerve, see Section 16.3).

3 *Parasympathetic nuclei*: These are the most laterally placed of the brain stem motor nuclei, equivalent to lateral horn cells of the spinal cord. They include Edinger–Westphal, superior and inferior salivatory, and the dorsal motor nucleus of the vagus.

Brain stem motor nuclei thus make up three interrupted columns: somatic motor, branchiomotor (special visceral motor) and parasympathetic (general visceral motor). This pattern is a useful basis for further study.

Table 2.2. Cranial nerve motor nuclei.

Nucleus	Position	Cranial nerve	Function
Somatic motor – voluntary			
Oculomotor	Upper midbrain	Oculomotor III	Eyeball movements: extrinsic ocular muscles
Trochlear	Lower midbrain	Trochlear IV	
Abducens	Pons	Abducens VI	
Hypoglossal	Medulla	Hypoglossal XII	Tongue muscles and movements
*Branchiomotor (special visceral motor) – voluntary**			
Trigeminal	Pons	Mandibular Vc (first)	Chewing, tensor tympani
Facial	Pons	Facial VII (second)	Facial expression, buccinator, stapedius
Nucleus ambiguus	Medulla	Glossopharyngeal IX (third)	Muscles of swallowing and phonation
		Vagus X, various branches (fourth)	
		Vagus (X), recurrent laryngeal (sixth)	

Table 2.2. (cont.)

Nucleus	Position	Cranial nerve	Function
Cervical accessory nucleus	Upper cervical spinal cord	Spinal accessory XI (see Section 16.3)	Sternocleidomastoid, trapezius
*Parasympathetic (general visceral motor) – involuntary**			
Edinger–Westphal	Midbrain	Oculomotor III	Ciliary muscle: lens accommodation, etc.; iris muscle: pupilloconstriction
Salivatory: superior	Pons	Facial VII	Secretomotor: lacrimal, nasal, palate, submandibular, sublingual glands
Salivatory: inferior	Upper medulla	Glossopharyngeal IX	Secretomotor: parotid gland
Dorsal motor of vagus	Medulla	Vagus X	Heart, foregut and midgut derivatives

* Cranial nerve with branchial arch.
** Cranial nerve conveying fibres from brain stem.

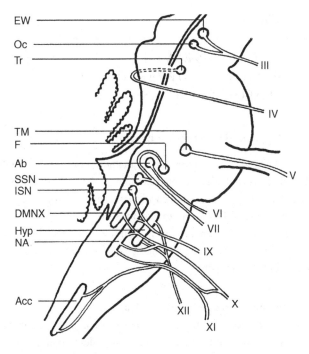

Fig. 2.1 Cranial nerve motor nuclei.
EW: Edinger–Westphal nucleus;
Oc: oculomotor nucleus;
Tr: trochlear nucleus;
TM: trigeminal motor nucleus;
Ab: abducens nucleus;
F: facial motor nucleus;
SSN: superior salivatory nucleus;
ISN: inferior salivatory nucleus;
DMNX: dorsal motor nucleus of X;
NA: nucleus ambiguus;
Hyp: hypoglossal nucleus;
Acc: lateral horn cells in cervical cord giving spinal roots of XI.

Chapter 3

CRANIAL NERVE MOTOR PATHWAYS: UPPER AND LOWER MOTOR NEURONS

3.1 Upper and lower motor neurons

Both somatic motor and branchiomotor nerves supply voluntary muscles. Pathways between motor cortex and muscles may be thought of as being arranged in two neuronal groups: upper motor neurons and lower motor neurons. Axons of upper motor neurons decussate before synapsing with lower motor neurons, so the right motor cortex controls the left side of the body, and vice versa – contralateral control.

Upper motor neurons: cortex to nucleus

For cranial nerves, cell bodies of upper motor neurons are in the head and neck area of the motor cortex. Axons descend, decussating just before synapsing with cell bodies of lower motor neurons which make up the motor nucleus of that cranial nerve. The term upper motor neurons is also used clinically to include fibres from other brain centres (e.g. parietal lobe, basal ganglia, cerebellum, reticular formation, midbrain, etc.) that connect with the lower motor neurons in the cranial nerve nucleus, thus influencing their activity.

Lower motor neurons: nucleus to muscle

Cell bodies of lower motor neurons form the brain stem nucleus. Axons leave the brain stem and pass in the cranial nerve to the destination. Thus, although most of the axon of the lower motor neuron is part of the peripheral nervous system, the cell body and first part of the axon is in the central nervous system.

3.2   Corticonuclear and corticobulbar

These terms describe the upper motor neuron pathways described above. They are often used interchangeably even though, since bulb means medulla, corticobulbar should be reserved for fibres passing to nuclei in the medulla.

3.3   Corticonuclear pathways (Fig. 3.1)

Frontal motor cortex

The head and neck area of the frontal motor cortex is found in the most lateral part of the precentral gyrus of the frontal lobe, immediately anterior to the central sulcus above the lateral fissure. It is supplied by branches of the middle cerebral artery. Its approximate surface marking is the pterion.

Corona radiata, internal capsule

Axons of upper motor neurons descend through the corona radiata and on to the genu of the internal capsule. The arterial supply of the internal capsule is from the medial and lateral striate branches of the middle cerebral artery.

Brain stem course

Axons of upper motor neurons descend through the central portions of the cerebral peduncles (crura) of the midbrain ventral to the substantia nigra and proceed as far as necessary, decussating just before synapsing on lower motor neuron cell bodies in the

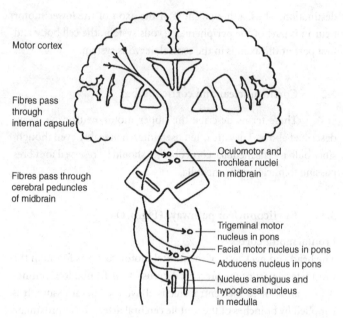

Motor cortex

Fibres pass through internal capsule

Fibres pass through cerebral peduncles of midbrain

Oculomotor and trochlear nuclei in midbrain

Trigeminal motor nucleus in pons

Facial motor nucleus in pons

Abducens nucleus in pons

Nucleus ambiguus and hypoglossal nucleus in medulla

Fig. 3.1 Corticonuclear pathways.

nuclei. The arterial supply of the brain stem is from branches of the basilar artery.

Blood supply
Blood vessels supplying the motor pathways are very important. A vascular lesion affecting any part of the pathway will have devastating effects. This is particularly so in the internal capsule since the same arteries supply not only motor but also neighbouring sensory pathways. A haemorrhage or an occlusion of the striate arteries is likely to affect a large area of the body leading to contralateral sensory and motor signs. This is often called a stroke.

3.4   Bilateral upper motor neuron control of III, IV, VI and part of VII

The pattern in the head and neck, as in the rest of the body, is that the motor cortex innervates contralateral motor nuclei. However, muscles which move the eyes, and the eyelids and forehead in association with eye movements, receive bilateral cortical innervation. The nuclei concerned are the oculomotor (III), trochlear (IV) and abducens (VI), and that portion of facial (VII) motor nucleus which innervates orbicularis oculi and frontalis. This must have evolved in association with, and for the protection of, the sense of sight by which means we seek sustenance and mates, and avoid danger.

There is limited bilateral control of the other voluntary motor nuclei as is evidenced by partial recovery of function in patients after a stroke.

3.5   Upper and lower motor neuron lesions

Lower motor neuron lesion: flaccidity, hyporeflexia, wasting, ipsilateral

If all lower motor neurons passing to a muscle are severed, the muscle will be completely paralyzed. It will be flaccid (atonic, hypotonic), it will not respond to reflexes (arreflexic, hyporeflexic) since no impulses reach it, and it will fairly quickly atrophy as a result of denervation. The injury and the paralysis are on the same side; they are ipsilateral with respect to each other.

Upper motor neuron lesion: spasticity, hyperreflexia, contralateral

If upper motor neurons to a muscle are severed, the ability to control and initiate movement in the muscle may be lost. However,

Table 3.1. Voluntary (somatic and branchiomotor) motor components of cranial nerves.

Nucleus	Type	Nerve	Muscles
Oculomotor *Midbrain*	Somatic *Preotic somites*	III Oculomotor	Levator palpebrae superioris, superior rectus, medial rectus, inferior rectus, inferior oblique
Trochlear *Midbrain*	Somatic *Preotic somites*	IV Trochlear	Superior oblique
Trigeminal motor *Pons for chewing*	Branchiomotor *first arch*	Vc Mandibular	Temporalis, masseter, digastric (anterior belly), mylohyoid, medial and lateral pterygoids, tensor palati, tensor tympani
Abducens *Pons*	Somatic *Preotic somites*	VI Abducens	Lateral rectus

Facial motor *Pons*	Branchiomotor *second arch*	VII Facial	Muscles of facial expression, buccinator, stapedius, occipitofrontalis, stylohyoid, digastric (posterior belly), platysma
Nucleus ambiguus *Medulla* for swallowing, phonation	Branchiomotor (see Section 16.3) *third arch* *fourth arch* *sixth arch*	IX Glossopharyngeal X Vagus, pharyngeal branches X Vagus, recurrent laryngeal XI Spinal accessory	Stylopharyngeus Muscles of pharynx Muscles of larynx Sternocleidomastoid, trapezius
Hypoglossal *Medulla*	Somatic *Occipital somites*	XII Hypoglossal	Intrinsic tongue muscles, hyoglossus, genioglossus, styloglossus

lower motor neurons are intact, and since some of the fibres to lower
motor neurons from elsewhere are inhibitory, other centres which
influence lower motor neurons, for example basal ganglia (Section
3.1), may cause an increase in muscle tone (hypertonic, spastic).
Also, reflexes are disinhibited (hyperreflexic, exaggerated). The
muscle will not become atrophied except through disuse. In this
case, since upper motor neurons decussate before synapsing with
cell bodies of lower motor neurons, the paralysis will be on the side
opposite to the site of the lesion; they are contralateral with respect
to each other. See Section 11.6 for consideration of facial nerve upper
and lower motor neuron lesions (UMNL and LMNL, respectively).

These characteristics of UMNL and LMNL are important. Get them
straight now! Study Table 3.1.

Chapter 4

CRANIAL NERVE SENSORY FIBRES, BRAIN STEM SENSORY NUCLEI AND TRACTS

Note: Sensory fibres carried by the olfactory, optic and vestibulo-cochlear nerves are not dealt with in this chapter. Consult Chapters 18, 20 and 23.

4.1 The basic plan of sensory systems

The basic sensory system consists of three neuronal groups:
- primary sensory neurons from receptor to central nucleus, with its cell body in a peripheral sensory ganglion;
- secondary sensory neurons from nucleus to diencephalon (usually the thalamus);
- tertiary sensory neurons from thalamus to cortex.

There are no synapses outside the brain and spinal cord: the first synapse is in the central nervous system (CNS) between primary and secondary sensory neurons.

Primary sensory neuron: receptor to sensory nucleus

This extends from peripheral receptor to CNS. The cell body is situated in a peripheral ganglion (dorsal root ganglion for spinal nerves) and the neuron is usually pseudounipolar, that is to say, it gives rise to a single axon which bifurcates into a peripheral process passing to the receptor, and a central process passing into the CNS. The cell body is thus both structurally and electrically out on a limb. The central process of the primary sensory neuron terminates by synapsing in a central nucleus which consists of cell bodies of the neuron next in the pathway …

Secondary sensory neurons: sensory nucleus to thalamus

The axons of these neurons ascend from the nucleus, which contains their cell bodies, to the contralateral thalamus (in the diencephalon), decussating soon after leaving the nucleus. In the thalamus, they synapse with the cell bodies of tertiary sensory neurons. (There are many other destinations of impulses from the nucleus, for example reticular nuclei and cerebellum, for the dissemination of information and its integration with other functions and systems.)

Tertiary sensory neurons: thalamus, internal capsule, cortex

Axons of tertiary sensory neurons extend from the thalamus to the appropriate area of sensory cortex and elsewhere, the neurons being known as thalamocortical neurons. These pass through the internal capsule. The principal sensory cortex for the head, to which somatic sensation is relayed by the thalamocortical neurons, is found on the lateral aspect of the parietal lobe behind the central sulcus and immediately above the lateral fissure. It is adjacent to the head and neck area of the motor cortex in the frontal lobe.

4.2   Sensory fibres in cranial nerves: somatic and visceral

Cranial nerves which transmit sensory fibres (other than I, II, VIII) are the trigeminal (V), facial (VII), glossopharyngeal (IX) and vagus (X). As described earlier (Section 1.6), sensory information may be classified as either somatic or visceral.

1 *Somatic sensory (somatosensory)*:

   Somatosensory fibres in cranial nerves convey pain, temperature, tactile and proprioceptive impulses from skin of the scalp, face, cheek and temple, oral cavity, teeth and gums, nasal cavity and sinuses, and temporomandibular joint and muscles. The trigeminal nerve is the principal somatosensory cranial nerve. All cranial nerve somatosensory fibres pass to the sensory nuclei of the trigeminal nerve, irrespective of the cranial nerve through which the fibres enter the brain stem.

2 *Visceral sensory*:

Visceral sensory fibres include taste fibres, fibres from the alimentary canal except the oral cavity, teeth and gums, and fibres from chemoreceptors and thoracoabdominal viscera. All cranial nerve visceral sensory fibres pass to the nucleus of the solitary tract, irrespective of the cranial nerve through which the fibres enter the brain stem.

4.3   Somatic sensation (Fig. 4.1)

All but a few somatosensory fibres from structures in the head are carried in the trigeminal (V) nerve. There are some somatosensory fibres in the vagus (X) nerve, and a few in the facial (VII) and glossopharyngeal (IX) nerves from the external ear. Cell bodies of primary sensory neurons are situated in the peripheral sensory ganglion (no synapses, remember) of the nerve through which they enter the brain stem.

Sensory ganglia for somatosensory fibres

Most somatic sensory fibres are carried in the trigeminal nerve: their cell bodies are in the trigeminal ganglion. The small number of somatosensory fibres in the vagus nerve (X) have cell bodies in the jugular (superior) vagal ganglion; those in the facial nerve (VII) have cell bodies in the geniculate ganglion; and those in the

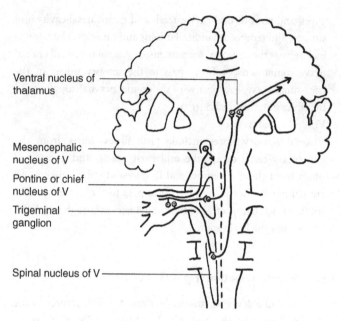

Fig. 4.1 Trigeminal (somatic) sensory system (e.g. cutaneous sensation), see also Fig. 5.1.

glossopharyngeal nerve (IX) have cell bodies in the superior glosso-pharyngeal ganglion.

Central connections of somatosensory fibres

Regardless of the nerve in which they are carried to the brain stem, within the CNS all somatosensory fibres pass to the sensory nuclei of the trigeminal nerve. This takes its name because the trigeminal nerve is its biggest single contributor. Table 4.1 lists somatic, sensory and visceral sensory ganglia and nuclei.

Table 4.1. Cranial nerve sensation, ganglia and nuclei.

	Source of stimulus	Ganglion	Nucleus and modality
Somatic sensory			
V	Oral and nasal cavities, teeth, TMJ, skin of anterior scalp, face, most of external ear	Trigeminal	Trigeminal: Spinal (pain, temperature)
VII	Small area of skin of external ear (sometimes)	Geniculate	Principal (tactile) mesencephalic
IX	Small area of skin of external ear (sometimes)	Superior glossopharyngeal	(proprioception from masticatory
X	Posterior skin of external ear	Jugular (superior) vagal	muscles – but see Section 4.4)

Table 4.1. (*cont.*)

	Source of stimulus	Ganglion	Nucleus and modality
Visceral sensory			
VII	Taste buds anterior tongue, palate	Geniculate	
IX	Mucosa of oropharynx; taste buds on posterior third of tongue; carotid body chemoreceptors and sinus	Petrosal (inferior) glossopharyngeal	Nucleus of solitary tract
X	Mucosa of hypopharynx, larynx; taste buds in epiglottic region and pharynx; aortic body chemoreceptors; sensation from thoracoabdominal viscera	Nodose (inferior) vagal	

	Source of stimulus	Ganglion	Nucleus and modality
Special sensory			
I	Olfactory receptors in olfactory epithelium	Bipolar cells of olfactory epithelium	Mitral cells of olfactory bulb
II	Rods and cones	Bipolar cells of retina	Lateral geniculate body
VIII	Organ of Corti	Spiral (cochlear)	Cochlear nuclei
VIII	Saccule, utricle, semicircular ducts	Vestibular	Vestibular nuclei

4.4   Somatic sensation: the trigeminal sensory nucleus and its projections (Fig. 4.1)

The trigeminal sensory nucleus has three parts, each for different modalities.

The principal or chief nucleus: tactile sensation

This is in the pons and receives the central processes of the primary sensory neurons transmitting tactile sensation. They synapse on cell bodies of secondary sensory neurons, the axons of which decussate and ascend in the trigeminal lemniscus to the contralateral thalamus (principally the ventral nucleus). A small proportion of fibres may also pass to the ipsilateral thalamus. Thalamocortical neurons pass as explained in Section 4.1.

The spinal tract and nucleus: pain and temperature sensation

This is so called because it extends down through the medulla into the cervical spinal cord. Caudally, it is in contact with the substantia gelatinosa of the dorsal horn of spinal grey matter which receives pain and temperature fibres of spinal nerves, and of which it can be considered a cranial extension. The spinal nucleus contains the cell bodies of secondary sensory pain and temperature neurons, the axons of which decussate and ascend in the trigeminal lemniscus to the contralateral thalamus, principally the ventromedial nuclear group. Thalamocortical neurons pass as explained in Section 4.1.

The mesencephalic nucleus: proprioceptive sensation, etc.

This is in the lower midbrain and receives impulses transmitting proprioceptive information from masticatory muscles, and deep pressure sensation from the teeth and gums. The mesencephalic nucleus is unique since it houses primary sensory nerve cell bodies which, for all other sensory fibres, would be in a peripheral ganglion. Although the details of its connections are not entirely clear, this arrangement allows other processes of the proprioceptive neurons to make connections with, for example, the motor nucleus of V, the salivatory nuclei, and the nucleus ambiguus – for chewing and swallowing (Section 13.1).

4.5   Visceral sensation: nucleus of the solitary tract

Clinically, this is less important than somatic sensation. Visceral sensory fibres enter the brain stem in the facial (VII), glossopharyngeal (IX) and vagus (X) nerves. Cell bodies of the primary sensory neurons are in the peripheral sensory ganglion (no synapses) of the nerve through which they enter the brain stem. Branches of the trigeminal (V) nerve are involved peripherally in the complex course of visceral sensory fibres, and visceral sensory fibres are often found in nerves which carry parasympathetic fibres in the opposite direction; they are described later in Chapter 17.

Sensory ganglia for visceral sensory fibres
Visceral sensory fibres entering the brain stem in the facial nerve (VII) have cell bodies in the geniculate ganglion; those in the glossopharyngeal nerve (IX) have cell bodies in the petrosal (inferior) glossopharyngeal ganglion; and those in the vagus nerve (X) have cell bodies in the nodose (inferior) vagal ganglion.

Central connections of visceral sensory fibres
Regardless of the nerve in which they are carried to the brain stem, within the CNS all visceral sensory fibres pass to the solitary tract and nucleus (nucleus tractus solitarius or NTS) in the medulla. Axons from the nucleus of the solitary tract pass rostrally by multisynaptic pathways, possibly bilateral, to the thalamus (ventral posteromedial nucleus), and thence probably to the insula and the uncus for connections with olfactory centres (Chapter 18).

INDIVIDUAL CRANIAL NERVES AND FUNCTIONAL CONSIDERATIONS

Chapter 5

SURVEY OF CRANIAL NERVES AND
INTRODUCTION TO PARTS II–V

In the following chapters we consider cranial nerves in groups concerned with their functions. These are, in no particular order, ingestion and chewing, cutaneous sensation, swallowing and speaking, autonomic function, taste and smell, and sight, hearing and balance.

The ingestion of food is dependent on opening the mouth. This is a function of the mandibular division of the trigeminal (Vc) and facial (VII) nerves: the mandibular opens the jaw and the facial parts the lips. The facial, mandibular and hypoglossal (XII) nerves are involved in taking the food into the mouth and closing the lips. Chewing is served by the same three nerves: in simple language, the facial nerve keeps the lips closed, the mandibular nerve moves the mandible for its mastication, and both facial and hypoglossal nerves maintain the food between the teeth. Also, the trigeminal senses its position and consistency, and regulates the force of contraction of the muscles, and both trigeminal and facial nerves are responsible for taste perception from the mouth. The trigeminal nerve also has another important function: the cutaneous sensation of the face and anterior scalp. It is, except for a small area of skin in the external ear, the only nerve concerned with this. So, the trigeminal, facial and hypoglossal nerves will be considered first.

After we eat and chew, we swallow. The motor components of swallowing are mainly the responsibility of the vagus (X) and glossopharyngeal (IX) nerves, with the hypoglossal (XII) nerve also initially involved. The vagus both innervates the muscles of swallowing, and senses, albeit unconsciously after the initial stages, its progress. It is also involved in phonation and speech which are related to swallowing in that many of the muscles and nerves are the same. These processes are aided by the glossopharyngeal nerve which, with the vagus, carries sensory information to the brain and participates in the perception of taste and the control of salivary secretions. The accessory nerve (XI) is an accessory to the vagus and so it too should be included in this group. After this, the loose ends of taste sensation and autonomic function may conveniently be tied up.

There is an embryological basis for studying the nerves in this order. The cranial end of the developing embryo is dominated by five pairs of structures which arise on either side of the primitive pharynx: these are the branchial (or pharyngeal) arches. Mandibular and facial movements and sensations are the functions of the first and second arches, of which the nerves are, respectively, the trigeminal and facial. Pharyngeal movements and sensations involved in swallowing are the concern of the third, fourth and sixth arches, and the nerves of these are the glossopharyngeal (third arch) and the vagus (fourth and sixth arches) (see Table 3.1 for more details).

This leaves the other main function of the head: the awareness of our surroundings. Our sense of smell is to a large extent linked with taste and basic physiological and psychological drives: it is therefore studied in connection with taste. Finally, vision, eye movements, balance and hearing are all interrelated and are considered together.

Thus, the cranial nerves are considered in the following order:

1 the trigeminal, facial and hypoglossal nerves (V, VII, XII);
2 the vagus, glossopharyngeal and accessory nerves (X, IX, XI);
3 autonomic function, taste sensation and olfaction (I);
4 vision and eye movements (II, III, IV, VI), and vestibular function and hearing (VIII).

Note

In Parts II–V the anatomical course of each nerve is usually described from its brain stem attachment outwards. However, each functional group of fibres is described according to the direction taken by the nerve impulse, motor fibres being described from central to peripheral, and sensory fibres from peripheral to central.

Some sections of the text are in note form. Within the text, important points are in bold print.

PART II

TRIGEMINAL, FACIAL AND HYPOGLOSSAL NERVES

Chapter 6

CUTANEOUS SENSATION
AND CHEWING

6.1   Think about it

If you were designing from scratch the cutaneous innervation
of the head and neck, it might strike you as logical to get down on
all fours like a quadruped and tilt your head back so that your face
was the most anterior part of you. In this position it makes sense
that the dorsal aspect of the neck and head should be supplied by
dorsal rami of spinal nerves, and the ventral aspect of the neck
and head (under the chin) by ventral rami. This leaves the entire
anterior aspect of the face, which, in a quadruped, goes first into
new environments, with a cutaneous nerve all to itself – the trigeminal. This is exactly how it is. All you have to do is remember that
because we are upright bipeds, the relative positions of the head
and trunk have changed as compared with the quadruped. Think
about it.

Sensory information from the face and scalp is carried back to the
trigeminal sensory nuclei (Section 4.4) in neurons with cell bodies
in the trigeminal ganglion (except for proprioceptive neurons), and
it is relayed to various centres within the brain. Examples of these
central connections can be illustrated by what happens when we wash
our face in the morning. Connections from the trigeminal nuclei
include those to:

1 the *sensory cortex and other cortical centres* for perception: we know
what we are doing;

2 the *limbic system*: a habit like this pleases us because our
   mothers conditioned us to do it when we were children (quite
   wrongly as it happens since soap is bad for the skin);
3 the *reticular formation*: it wakes us up;
4 the *hypothalamus*: vasoconstriction or vasodilatation, according
   to the temperature of the water.

The second and third divisions of the trigeminal innervate the
roof and floor of the mouth, so it will not surprise you to learn that
they are involved not only with cutaneous sensation but also with
sensation in the oral cavity and with movements of the mandible.

6.2   Motor aspects of ingestion and chewing

The motor aspects of ingestion and chewing are:
- *Depression of mandible*: lateral pterygoid, mylohyoid, anterior
  digastric (mandibular nerve (Vc)).
- *Parting of lips*: inhibition of orbicularis oris (facial nerve (VII)).
- *Removal of food from fork*.
- *Closing lips*: orbicularis oris (facial nerve (VII)).
- *Elevation of mandible* (occlusion): masseter, temporalis, medial
  pterygoid (mandibular nerve (Vc)).
- *Tongue movements* (hypoglossal nerve (XII)).
- *Mandibular movements*: temporalis, masseter, pterygoids, etc.
  (mandibular nerve (Vc)).
- *Maintenance of bolus between teeth* (in occlusal plane):
  - Buccinator (facial nerve (VII)).
  - Tongue (hypoglossal nerve (XII)).

In a baby before weaning, the buccinator (VII) and the tongue (XII)
are the principal muscles of sustenance producing the necessary
sucking forces. Damage to VII in infants, for example birth injuries,
will impair feeding (see Facial nerve injury in babies in Section 11.7).

6.3   Sensory aspects of ingestion and chewing

Sensory functions of the mandibular nerve are important in sensing how hard the masticatory muscles must contract in order to chew effectively without damaging the teeth and gums. These muscles, masseter in particular, exert great force. This proprioceptive information is carried to the mesencephalic nucleus of the trigeminal nerve (Section 4.4) and thence to other brain stem nuclei.

The consistency of the food is sensed by branches of the mandibular nerve and when this is judged satisfactory, the bolus is propelled backwards on to the posterior (glossopharyngeal) portion of the tongue and swallowing begins. Once the bolus has passed the posterior portion of the tongue, the process is irreversible or, at any rate, reversible only with a great deal of coughing and spluttering.

6.4   Salivation and taste

Parasympathetic fibres in cranial nerves are secretomotor: they are concerned with the stimulation of secretions from the submandibular, sublingual, parotid and minor palatal salivary glands. These impulses originate in the superior and inferior salivatory nuclei and pass to the glands through branches of the facial and glossopharyngeal nerves, and, peripherally, the trigeminal. They are considered in more detail in Part IV. Impulses from the sensory nuclei of the trigeminal nerve pass to the salivatory nuclei to influence salivary production.

Branches of the trigeminal and facial nerves also transmit taste sensation fibres from the anterior portion of the tongue and the oral mucosa to the solitary tract and nucleus. Taste is considered separately in Part IV.

Chapter 7

THE TRIGEMINAL NERVE (V)

7.1 Functions

The trigeminal nerve transmits sensation from the skin of the anterior part of the head, the oral and nasal cavities, the teeth and the meninges. It has three divisions (ophthalmic, maxillary and mandibular) subsequently treated as separate nerves. Its mandibular division also carries motor fibres to muscles used in chewing.

7.2 Attachment, course, divisions (Fig. 7.1)

- Attached to lateral aspect of pons, near middle cerebellar peduncle.
- Passes below tentorium cerebelli, to middle cranial fossa.
- Trigeminal (sensory) ganglion in depression on temporal bone.
- Splits into ophthalmic (Va), maxillary (Vb) and mandibular (Vc).

7.3 Trigeminal ganglion

- It contains cell bodies of primary sensory neurons in all three divisions of trigeminal nerve, except those of proprioceptive neurons (see Chapter 4).
- It is partially surrounded by cerebrospinal fluid in recess of sub-arachnoid space: trigeminal, or Meckel's, cave.

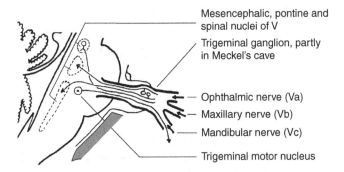

Fig. 7.1 Trigeminal nerve (see also Fig. 4.1).

7.4   Clinical notes

1 *Shingles and varicella-zoster*

   The trigeminal ganglion, as any sensory ganglion, may be the site of infection by the herpes zoster virus causing shingles, a painful vesicular eruption in the sensory distribution of the nerve. The virus may have been latent in the ganglion following chickenpox (varicella).

2 *Trigeminal neuralgia*

   This is severe pain in the distribution of the trigeminal nerve or one of its branches, the cause often being unknown. It may require partial destruction of the ganglion.

Chapter 8

THE OPHTHALMIC NERVE (Va)

8.1   Functions

The ophthalmic nerve transmits sensory fibres from the eyeball, the skin of the upper face and anterior scalp, the lining of the upper part of the nasal cavity and air cells, and the meninges of the anterior cranial fossa. Some of its branches also convey parasympathetic fibres (see below).

8.2   Origin, course and branches (Fig. 8.1)

- originates from trigeminal ganglion in middle cranial fossa passes anteriorly through lateral wall of cavernous sinus.
- divides into three branches: **frontal** (largest), nasociliary and lacrimal (smallest) which pass through superior orbital fissure to orbit.

Frontal nerve (frontal sinus, and skin of forehead and scalp):
- Passes immediately below frontal bone and divides into **supraorbital** (larger, lateral) and **supratrochlear** (medial) nerves.
- Supraorbital nerve in supraorbital notch (with branch of ophthalmic artery) turns up to supply skin of forehead and scalp (back to vertex).
- **Nerves and vessels in scalp are superficial to aponeurosis.**

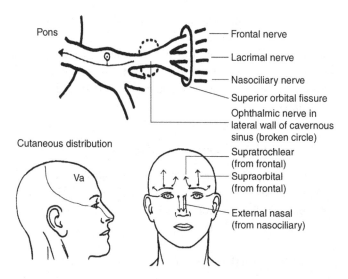

Fig. 8.1 Ophthalmic nerve.

Nasociliary nerve (eyeball, upper part of nasal cavity, and ethmoidal and sphenoidal air cells, anterior nasal skin, and meninges):

• Passes through superior orbital fissure within common tendinous ring.

• Long and short ciliary nerves to eyeball to innervate ocular structures including cornea. Short ciliary nerves contain parasympathetic impulses from ciliary ganglion (Chapter 17). Long and short ciliary nerves also contain sympathetic fibres (Chapter 19).

• Anterior ethmoidal nerve gives sensory fibres to meninges of anterior cranial fossa, enters nasal cavity. Supplies upper part of nasal cavity, and sphenoid and ethmoid air cells. Continues as external nasal nerve supplying cutaneous sensation to anterior aspect and tip of nose.

Lacrimal nerve (lacrimal gland, and small area of adjacent skin and conjunctiva: not important):
- Superior orbital fissure: lateral to (outside) common tendinous ring.
- Joined by postganglionic parasympathetic fibres from pterygopalatine ganglion. These are distributed to lacrimal gland (see Section 17.3).

8.3   Nerve fibres: central connections

Somatic sensory fibres: sensory nuclei of trigeminal nerve.

Present in all branches. Axons pass centrally with cell bodies in trigeminal ganglion. Central axonal processes pass to pons and trigeminal sensory nuclei (Section 4.4).

Parasympathetic pathways: not important (see Chapter 17).

8.4   Clinical notes

1 *Corneal reflex*
   When the cornea is touched, usually with a wisp of cotton wool, the subject blinks. This tests V and VII. The nerve impulses pass thus: cornea, nasociliary nerve, Va, principal sensory nucleus of V, brain stem interneurons, facial motor nucleus, VII, orbicularis oculi muscle. Note that the reflex does not test vision or eye movements.
2 *Supraorbital injuries*
   Trauma to the supraorbital margin may damage the supraorbital and/or supratrochlear nerves causing sensory loss in the scalp.
3 *Ethmoid tumours*
   Malignant tumours of the mucous lining of the ethmoid air cells may expand into the orbits, damaging branches of Va, particularly the ethmoidal nerves. This may lead to displacement of the

orbital contents causing proptosis and squint, and sensory loss over the anterior nasal skin.

4 *Nasal fractures*

Trauma to the nose may damage the external nasal nerve as it becomes superficial. Sensory loss of the skin down to the tip of the nose may result.

5 *Bilateral cleft lip and palate*

In this condition, the central part of the upper lip together with that part of the palate posterior to it which bears the upper incisors are isolated from surrounding areas. Branches of the maxillary nerve are thus denied access. The isolated area of palate and lip in these cases are supplied by Va through its external nasal branch which enters from above. In a unilateral cleft, Vb of one side is able to innervate the area in an asymmetric fashion.

8.5   Clinical testing

1 Test corneal reflex (see above).
2 Test skin sensation of forehead and anterior scalp.

Chapter 9

THE MAXILLARY NERVE (Vb)

9.1 Functions

The maxillary nerve transmits sensory fibres from the skin of the face between the palpebral fissure and the mouth, from the nasal cavity and sinuses, and from the maxillary teeth.

At its origin it contains only sensory fibres. Some of its branches transmit postganglionic parasympathetic fibres from the pterygopalatine ganglion which pass to the lacrimal, nasal and palatine glands (see Section 17.3), and others convey taste (visceral sensory) fibres from the palate to the nucleus of the solitary tract (see Section 17.4).

9.2 Origin, course and branches (Fig. 9.1)

- originates from trigeminal ganglion in middle cranial fossa;
- passes in lower part of lateral wall of cavernous sinus;
- meningeal branch (middle cranial fossa – sensory);
- foramen rotundum, to;
- pterygopalatine fossa which divides into main branches, infra-orbital and zygomatic, and gives other branches to nose, palate and upper teeth.

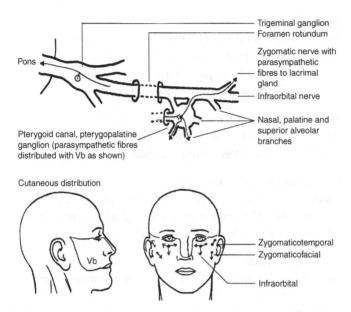

Fig. 9.1 Maxillary nerve.

Infraorbital nerve – infraorbital skin, upper lip

Passes anteriorly between orbit and maxillary antrum in infraorbital groove. Twigs to mucosal lining of **maxillary antrum**.

Emerges at infraorbital foramen to supply **skin over cheek and upper lip**.

Zygomatic nerve – zygomatic skin

Enters orbit through inferior orbital fissure. Two small cutaneous branches penetrate zygoma: zygomaticofacial and zygomaticotemporal. Conveys postganglionic parasympathetic fibres from pterygopalatine ganglion to lacrimal gland (see Chapter 17).

Nasal branches
Pass medially from pterygopalatine fossa through sphenopalatine foramen into nasal cavity. Supply nasal cavity and sinuses. Branches also convey postganglionic parasympathetic fibres from pterygopalatine ganglion to nasal glands (see Chapter 17).

Superior alveolar (dental) nerves
Branches of infraorbital and palatine nerves pass directly through maxilla to **maxillary teeth, gums and sinus**.

Greater and lesser palatine nerves
Hard and soft palate sensation. Branches also convey postganglionic parasympathetic fibres from pterygopalatine ganglion to minor salivary glands in the palatal mucosa (see Chapter 17).

Pharyngeal branch
Passes posteriorly to contribute to sensory supply of nasopharynx.

9.3   Nerve fibres: central connections

Somatic sensory fibres: sensory nuclei of trigeminal nerve
Present in all branches of maxillary nerve. Axons pass centrally with cell bodies in trigeminal ganglion. Central processes pass to pons and trigeminal sensory nuclei (Section 4.4). *Note: sensory fibres traversing pterygopalatine ganglion, for example those from palate and nose, do not synapse there.*

Taste (visceral sensory) fibres: nucleus of solitary tract
From scattered taste buds on palate. Axons ascend in palatine nerves, through pterygopalatine ganglion (no synapse), pterygoid canal, greater petrosal and facial nerve (cell bodies in geniculate ganglion). Central processes enter brain stem through nervus intermedius, passing to nucleus of solitary tract (see Chapter 17).

Parasympathetic fibres: superior salivatory nucleus
Superior salivatory nucleus, nervus intermedius, VII, lacrimal, nasal and palatal glands (see Chapter 17).

9.4   Clinical notes

1 *Infraorbital injuries: malar fractures*
  Trauma to infraorbital margin may cause sensory loss of infra-orbital skin.
2 *Maxillary sinus infections*
  Infections of the maxillary sinus may cause infraorbital pain or may cause referred pain to other structures supplied by Vb (e.g. upper teeth).
3 *Maxillary antrum tumours*
  Malignant tumours of the mucous lining of the maxillary antrum may expand into the orbit, damaging branches of Vb, particularly the infraorbital. This may lead to anaesthesia over the facial skin. The orbital contents may also be displaced causing proptosis and/or a squint.
4 *Maxillary teeth abscesses*
  The roots of the maxillary teeth (especially the second molars) are intimately related to the maxillary sinus. Root abscesses are painful.
5 *Hay fever*
  This is usually allergic, but the symptoms could be produced by involvement of parasympathetic "fellow travellers" with the maxillary nerve (see Section 17.3).

9.5   Clinical testing

Test skin sensation of lower eyelid, cheek and upper lip.

Chapter 10

THE MANDIBULAR NERVE (Vc)

10.1 Functions

The mandibular nerve is a mixed sensory and motor nerve. It transmits sensory fibres from the skin over the mandible, side of the cheek and temple, the oral cavity and contents, the external ear, the tympanic membrane and temporomandibular joint (TMJ). It also supplies the meninges of the cranial vault.

It is motor to the eight muscles derived from the first branchial arch:

- temporalis, masseter
- medial, lateral pterygoids
- mylohyoid, anterior belly of digastric
- tensor tympani, tensor palati

As an aid to memory, note the four groups of two: tensors, pterygoids, big muscles and the last two in the floor of the mouth.

Some of its distal branches also convey parasympathetic secretomotor fibres to the salivary glands, and taste fibres from the anterior portion of the tongue.

10.2 Origin, course and branches (Fig. 10.1)

- From trigeminal ganglion in middle cranial fossa.
- Foramen ovale.
- Infratemporal fossa with four main branches: **inferior alveolar, lingual, auriculotemporal, buccal**.
- Motor branches to muscles listed above.

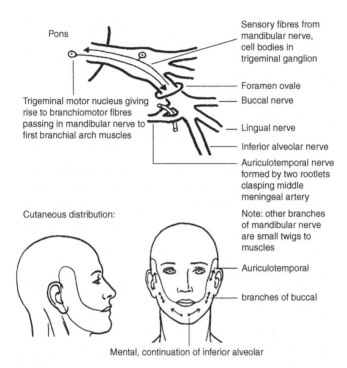

Pons

Sensory fibres from
mandibular nerve,
cell bodies in
trigeminal ganglion

Foramen ovale

Buccal nerve

Trigeminal motor nucleus giving
rise to branchiomotor fibres
passing in mandibular nerve to
first branchial arch muscles

Lingual nerve

Inferior alveolar nerve

Auriculotemporal nerve
formed by two rootlets
clasping middle
meningeal artery

Cutaneous distribution:

Note: other branches
of mandibular nerve
are small twigs to
muscles

Auriculotemporal

branches of buccal

Mental, continuation of inferior alveolar

Fig. 10.1 Mandibular nerve.

Inferior alveolar nerve: lower teeth, skin, mylohyoid, digastric

Enters mandibular foramen, supplies lower teeth. Just before mandibular foramen, gives off nerve to mylohyoid and anterior belly
of digastric, running in groove on medial aspect of mandible.
Mental nerve emerges from mental foramen on anterior aspect of
mandible to supply skin.

Lingual nerve: tongue sensation

**Lingual nerve immediately below and medial to the third lower
molar (wisdom) tooth.** Passes forwards in floor of mouth, winding

around submandibular duct. Supplies anterior tongue, gums. Conveys parasympathetic fibres from superior salivatory nucleus, and taste fibres to VII; these pass between lingual nerve and VII in chorda tympani (see Chapter 17).

Auriculotemporal nerve: skin of temple, TMJ, external ear
Arises beneath foramen ovale by two rootlets on either side of middle meningeal artery. Passes above parotid gland, between TMJ and external auditory meatus to emerge on side of head. Ascends close to superficial temporal artery. Supplies **TMJ**, parotid fascia, skin of temple, most of **skin of external auditory meatus and tympanic membrane**. For short distance between foramen ovale and parotid gland it conveys parasympathetic fibres for innervation of parotid gland (see Chapter 17).

Buccal nerve: skin and mucosa of cheek
Supplies sensory fibres to skin and mucosa of cheek (it does NOT supply buccinator (see Section 11.3)).

Muscular branches: temporal nerves to temporalis, and other muscular twigs.

Meningeal branches: Small twigs re-enter middle cranial fossa through foramen ovale, and other foramina, to supply meninges.

10.3   The first branchial arch

The mandibular nerve is the main nerve of the first branchial arch (the maxillary nerve also contributes). The first branchial arch gives rise to: a precursor of the mandible (Meckel's cartilage), the spine of the sphenoid, the sphenomandibular ligament, the malleus and incus, and the eight muscles listed above (see Section 10.1). Arterial components of the first arch degenerate.

10.4   Nerve fibres: central connections

Somatic sensory fibres: sensory nuclei of the trigeminal nerve
Axons pass centrally with cell bodies in trigeminal ganglion.
Central processes to pons and trigeminal sensory nuclei (see
Section 4.4).

Branchiomotor fibres: trigeminal motor nucleus
Trigeminal motor nucleus in pons, axons to mandibular nerve and
eight muscles of first branchial arch (see above).

Visceral sensory (taste) fibres: nucleus of the solitary tract
Taste fibres from anterior portion of tongue pass in lingual nerve,
chorda tympani and facial nerve. Cell bodies in geniculate ganglion.
Central processes to nucleus of solitary tract (see Section 4.5).

Parasympathetic pathways: salivatory nuclei
Branches of mandibular nerve convey parasympathetic impulses to
submandibular, sublingual and parotid glands (see Chapter 17).

10.5   Clinical notes

1 *Lingual nerve*
   Careless extractions of the third lower molar (wisdom) tooth,
   abscesses of its root, etc., or fractures of the angle of the
   mandible may all damage the lingual nerve. This may result not
   only in loss of somatic sensation from the anterior portion of the
   tongue, but also loss of taste sensation and parasympathetic
   function.
2 *Inferior alveolar nerve and inferior alveolar nerve block*
   Trauma to the mandible may damage or tear the inferior alveolar nerve in the mandibular canal leading to sensory loss distal to

the lesion. Local anaesthesia of the inferior alveolar nerve is com-
monly performed for dental procedures. Injection of local anaes-
thetics into the oral mucosa on the medial side of the mandible
can also involve the nearby lingual nerve, thus affecting the
tongue and inside of the mouth. In wisdom teeth extractions, the
buccal nerve may also be anaesthetized leading to numbness of
the cheek.

3 *Mumps*

Mumps is inflammation of the parotid gland causing tension in
the parotid capsule which is innervated by the auriculotemporal
nerve. It gives both local tenderness and referred earache. It is
very uncomfortable.

4 *Submandibular duct*

The intimate relationship between the submandibular duct and
the lingual nerve is significant in duct infections and surgery. Submandibular stones are not uncommon because of the mucous
secretions. If the lingual nerve were damaged there would be
sensory loss, both somatic and taste, in the anterior portion of
the tongue.

5 *Referred pain to the ear*

Disease of the TMJ or swelling of the parotid gland may cause
earache because of referred pain. Also, pain from the lower teeth,
oral cavity and tongue may be referred to the ear. Beware of
patients with cotton wool in the external auditory meatus –
check in the mouth for the disease!

6 *Superficial temporal artery biopsy*

The auriculotemporal nerve accompanies the superficial temporal artery on the temple. In cases of temporal arteritis, the nerve
is anaesthetized so that the overlying skin can be incised to
obtain a biopsy of the artery.

10.6   Clinical testing

1 Sensory: Test skin sensation of chin and lower lip.
2 Motor: feel contractions of masseter, temporalis. Open jaw
  against resistance (pterygoids, mylohyoid, anterior digastric).

Chapter 11

THE FACIAL NERVE (VII)

11.1 Functions

The facial nerve supplies the muscles of facial expression.
Its other functions are:
- taste sensation from the anterior portion of the tongue and oral cavity;
- parasympathetic secretomotor function of the salivary, lacrimal, nasal and palatine glands.

11.2 Origin

- It originates from **cerebellopontine angle** – lateral part of pontomedullary junction.
- Two adjacent roots: **motor root** (larger, more medial); nervus intermedius (smaller, more lateral) – so called because it is found between two larger nerves (main root of VII and VIII). Nervus intermedius conveys parasympathetic and sensory fibres and may be part of VIII initially.

11.3 Course and branches (Figs 11.1 and 11.2)

Intracranial course and branches (Fig. 11.1):
- From cerebellopontine angle, crosses posterior cranial fossa, enters **internal acoustic meatus** (IAM; with VIII).
- Nervus intermedius joins main root of facial nerve in IAM.

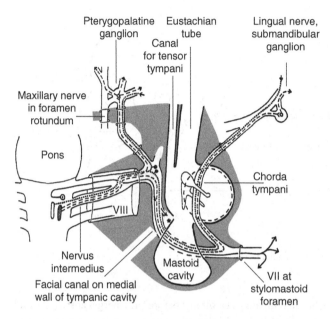

Fig. 11.1 Facial nerve (intracranial). ○——▸ : branchiomotor fibres from facial motor nucleus to muscles of facial expression, stapedius, etc.; ▮------▸ : parasympathetic preganglionic fibres from superior salivatory nucleus; ▯--○-◂--- : nucleus of solitary tract receiving visceral sensory fibres, cell bodies in geniculate (sensory) ganglion; * to stapedius; stippled area represents bone.

- Geniculate ganglion is deep in IAM: this houses cell bodies of sensory fibres (no synapses) in VII. Nerve turns posteriorly into:
- Facial canal running posteriorly along medial wall of tympanic (middle ear) cavity, and gives branch to stapedius (attached to stapes);

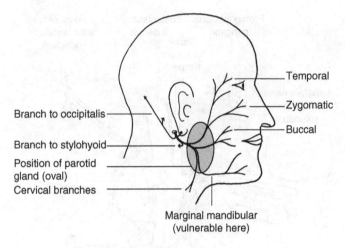

Fig. 11.2 Facial nerve (extracranial).

- Chorda tympani given off just before VII emerges at stylomastoid foramen; this passes anteriorly across tympanic membrane into infratemporal fossa where it joins lingual nerve;
- Emerges at stylomastoid foramen.

Extracranial course and branches (Fig. 11.2)
- Outside stylomastoid foramen, small branches of VII supply occipital belly of occipitofrontalis, stylohyoid and posterior belly of digastric, and a variable amount of cutaneous sensation from skin of external auditory meatus.
- Nerve enters **parotid gland** where it forms intricate plexus. **Branches of VII are superficial in the gland**.
- Five groups of branches emerge superficially from anterior border of parotid gland: temporal, zygomatic, buccal, mandibular and

cervical. These supply **muscles of facial expression** including orbicularis oculi, orbicularis oris, buccinator and platysma.

The most important thing about the intracranial course of VII is its relationship to the middle ear. The most important thing about the extracranial course is its relationship to the parotid gland.

11.4   The second branchial arch, otic vesicle and facial nerve

The facial nerve is the nerve of the second branchial arch which gives rise to part of the hyoid bone, the styloid process, the stylohyoid ligament, the stapes and the muscles listed in Section 11.3: the muscles of facial expression (which migrate into superficial layers), stylohyoid, posterior belly of digastric, occipitofrontalis and stapedius. Arterial components of the second arch degenerate.

The facial nerve develops in association with the otic vesicle, and with the first branchial pouch (endodermal) and the first branchial cleft (ectodermal) which lie between the first and second arches. This accounts for the intimate relationship of the facial nerve with the derivatives of these structures: the inner, middle and external ears.

11.5   Nerve fibres: central connections

Branchiomotor fibres: facial motor nucleus

Facial motor nucleus in pons, axons pass dorsally, then loop ventrally around abducens (VI) nucleus, causing elevation (facial colliculus) on floor of fourth ventricle. (It has been suggested that this peculiar course may be a result of the developmental phenomenon of neurobiotaxis in which a cell body migrates towards the greatest density of stimuli.)

Preganglionic parasympathetic fibres: superior salivatory nucleus

Superior salivatory nucleus in lower pons, preganglionic axons into nervus intermedius and VII. Some pass to pterygopalatine ganglion (synapse) for lacrimal, nasal and palatine glands. Some enter chorda tympani and pass to submandibular ganglion (synapse) for submandibular and sublingual glands (see Chapter 17). *Parasympathetic fibres not present in extracranial portion.*

Visceral sensory (taste) fibres: solitary tract and nucleus

Taste fibres from anterior portion of tongue, through lingual nerve to chorda tympani, VII. Cell bodies in geniculate ganglion. Central processes pass in nervus intermedius to solitary tract and nucleus. Taste fibres from palate pass through pterygoid canal and greater petrosal nerve to facial nerve, then as above. *Taste fibres not present in extracranial portion of VII.*

Somatic sensory fibres: sensory nuclei of the trigeminal nerve

From small and variable area of skin in region of ear, and external aspect of tympanic membrane, fibres join facial nerve just outside stylomastoid foramen. Cell bodies in geniculate ganglion. Central processes pass to sensory nuclei of trigeminal nerve.

11.6   Upper and lower motor neuron lesions of the facial nerve

In upper motor neuron (UMN) lesions of the facial nerve, the forehead and orbicularis oculi muscles are largely spared. This is because there is bilateral cortical control of the upper facial muscles, and so if corticonuclear fibres on one side of the brain are interrupted (e.g. in the internal capsule) those of the other side are unaffected. For the lower facial muscles this is not so: the normal pattern prevails with only contralateral control.

UMN lesion of the facial nerve

The facial motor nucleus is divided into two parts:

1 that for upper facial muscles (orbicularis oculi and frontalis);
2 that for lower facial muscles.

The lower motor neuron (LMN) cell bodies in (1) receive UMNs from both cerebral motor cortices, ipsilateral *as well as* the usual contralateral. LMNs in (2) do not: they receive only the customary contralateral innervation. Thus, a unilateral UMN lesion of the fibres supplying (1) will *not* result in complete functional loss since UMN input is also present from the other side. However, for the lower part of the face, there would be no sparing since the UMN input comes only from the contralateral cortex. This is usually obvious since when facial muscles lose their tone, facial wrinkles also disappear.

The significance of this has been pointed out in Section 3.4. It is associated with eye movements and eye protection.

LMN lesion of the facial nerve – facial palsy

An LMN lesion, whether of cell bodies in the facial motor nucleus, or of any part of the peripheral course of the facial nerve, intracranial or extracranial, would result in a complete ipsilateral LMN lesion of the facial nerve, irrespective of which part of the facial nucleus was involved. The bilateral UMN innervation to the upper part of the face would be of no significance since the lesion affects the more distal LMN. An LMN lesion of the facial nerve is called a facial palsy.

11.7   Other clinical notes

1 *Parotid disease*
   Parotid tumours, trauma or surgery may damage branches of
   the facial nerve. This would result in an ipsilateral facial palsy
   with wasting and functional loss. It would be unlikely to recover.

2 *Stapedius: hyperacusis*
   Dysfunction of the smallest muscle supplied by the facial nerve
   can cause a distressing symptom. Stapedius dampens the movements of the ossicular chain and if it is inactive, sounds will be
   distorted and echoing. This is hyperacusis. See also Stapedius
   paralysis: hyperacusis in Section 23.5.

3 *Bell's palsy*
   This is a facial palsy, usually of unknown aetiology. It has been
   suggested that vascular spasm of the arteries in the facial canal
   supplying the nerve might be responsible, or inflammation and
   swelling of the nerve within the bony canal.

4 *Corneal reflex*
   A test of the ophthalmic and facial nerves (see Corneal reflex in
   Section 8.4).

5 *The marginal mandibular branch of the facial nerve*
   This branch passes on or just below the lower margin of the
   mandible. It is superficial even to the palpable facial arterial
   pulse and is thus liable to injury. Section of this nerve would
   result in paralysis of the muscles of the corner of the mouth:
   drooling would occur.

6 *Facial nerve injury in babies*
   As the mastoid process is rudimentary at birth, the facial
   nerve is more easily damaged in babies. Birth injuries, or other
   trauma, can therefore cause an ipsilateral facial palsy. This is
   serious since buccinator, supplied by VII, is necessary for sucking
   (feeding).

7 *Cerebellopontine angle tumours*

Tumours in this region would cause signs and symptoms of damage to the facial and vestibulocochlear nerves and cerebellar signs. These include facial palsy, deafness, vertigo and poor coordination.

8 *Acoustic neuroma*

This is a tumour of Schwann cells on the vestibular nerve in the IAM. Since the tumour grows within a bony canal it may compress the facial and vestibulocochlear nerves causing a particular type of deafness (nerve deafness) and an ipsilateral facial palsy.

9 *Brain stem lesions*

The relationship between the nucleus of the abducens nerve and the axons of the facial nerve means that a brain stem lesion may cause a paralysis of the facial nerve in association with a paralysis of the ipsilateral lateral rectus muscle of the eye.

10 *Geniculate herpes, Ramsay Hunt syndrome*

The herpes zoster virus may lie dormant in the geniculate ganglion (after an attack of chickenpox) and at some later stage cause a vesicular eruption in the skin around the external auditory meatus supplied by the facial nerve. There may also be signs on the anterior portion of the tongue as a result of taste fibres with cell bodies in the geniculate ganglion. The inflammation may spread to involve the motor fibres in the facial nerve. A LMN lesion arising from this cause is known as the Ramsay Hunt syndrome.

11.8   Clinical testing

1 Observe the face. Normal facial movements (lips, eyelids, emotions) and the presence of normal facial skin creases indicate an intact nerve.
2 Test strength by trying to force apart tightly closed eyelids. This should be difficult.
3 Test corneal reflex (see Corneal reflex in Section 8.4).

Chapter 12

THE HYPOGLOSSAL NERVE (XII)

12.1   Function

The hypoglossal nerve supplies the muscles of the tongue.
Movements of the tongue are important in chewing, in the initial
stages of swallowing and in speech. It also conveys fibres from C1
which innervate the strap muscles.

12.2   Origin, course and branches (Fig. 12.1)

The hypoglossal nerve (XII):

- Originates from medulla by vertical series of rootlets between
  pyramid and olive (see Section 1.4). Hypoglossal (condylar) canal
  in occipital bone.
- Receives motor fibres from C1 and descends to submandibular
  region.
- Turns forwards, lateral to external carotid artery, **hooking
  beneath origin of occipital artery**. Passes lateral to hyoglossus
  and enters tongue from below.
- Gives descendens hypoglossi to ansa cervicalis carrying fibres from
  C1 to strap muscles; other C1 fibres remain with XII to supply
  geniohyoid.
- Supplies **intrinsic muscles of tongue**, hyoglossus, genioglossus and
  styloglossus.

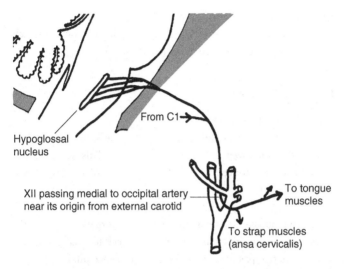

Fig. 12.1 Hypoglossal nerve.

12.3   Occipital somites

The hypoglossal nerve is the nerve of occipital somites. The motor nucleus is adjacent to, and equivalent to, ventral horn cells in C1 segment of the spinal cord, some axons from which run with the hypoglossal nerve for a short distance (see above).

12.4   Nerve fibres and central connections

Somatic motor fibres: hypoglossal nucleus

Hypoglossal nucleus in medulla close to the midline: somatic motor nuclear column (like nuclei of III, IV, VI). Axons pass directly to tongue muscles.

Sensory fibres: uncertain

A few sensory fibres from sternocleidomastoid and trapezius. Cell bodies (unusually) scattered along length of nerve.

12.5   Clinical notes

1 *Hypoglossal nerve lesions*

 Damage to the hypoglossal nerve in the neck would result in an ipsilateral lower motor neuron lesion. This would cause the protruded tongue to deviate to the side of the lesion (see Section 12.6).

2 *Carotid artery surgery, block dissection of neck*

 The hypoglossal nerve is vulnerable in surgery (e.g. carotid endarterectomy, block dissection of the neck for malignant disease) where it passes under the origin of the occipital artery.

3 *Bulbar and pseudobulbar palsy*

 For details refer to Section 13.3.

12.6   Clinical testing

1 Ask the patient to protrude tongue. If it deviates to one side, then the nerve of that side is damaged – the tongue is pushed to the paralysed side by muscles of the functioning side.

2 Ask patient to push tongue into cheek, then palpate cheek to feel tone and strength of tongue muscles.

PART III

GLOSSOPHARYNGEAL, VAGUS AND ACCESSORY NERVES

Chapter 13

SWALLOWING AND SPEAKING, BULBAR PALSY, PSEUDOBULBAR PALSY, BROCA'S AREA

13.1 Swallowing

When food or drink passes on to the posterior part of the tongue, the muscles supplied by the nucleus ambiguus through the vagus (X) and glossopharyngeal (IX) nerves propel it backwards and downwards into the hypopharynx, thence through the cricopharyngeal sphincter to the oesophagus. The nasopharynx is closed by the palatal muscles (X, Vc), and the Eustachian tube opens (X). The laryngeal orifice is reduced in size largely as a result of elevation of the entire laryngeal skeleton by all the muscles attaching to it from above, and the cricopharyngeal sphincter opens (X). The tongue muscles (XII) also have an important role in these actions. Most of the muscles of the pharynx are supplied in one way or another by the nucleus ambiguus through the vagus (it is unnecessary to bother with individual pharyngeal muscles).

Sensation from this region is conveyed through the pharyngeal plexus, the glossopharyngeal (posterior tongue, oropharynx) and vagus (hypopharynx) nerves, to the nucleus of the solitary tract.

13.2 Speaking

Noise production: phonation
The vocal cords create the narrow slit through which air is directed to make a sound, much as in an oboe, recorder or organ pipe.

Muscles which move the cords are supplied by the recurrent laryngeal nerve (X).

Making the noise intelligible: articulation

The pharyngeal muscles (X), the tongue (XII), the muscles of facial expression (VII), mandibular movements (Vc) and the palate (X, V) all modify the crude noise produced by the larynx to create speech.

Pitch

Pitch is modulated principally by tensing (cricothyroid) and relaxing (vocalis) the vocal cords. All movements of the vocal cords are controlled by the nucleus ambiguus through the superior and recurrent laryngeal nerves (X). It is unnecessary to learn individual laryngeal muscles or their attachments; it is enough to know that they are all innervated by the nucleus ambiguus. Lesions affecting the nucleus ambiguus lead to profound swallowing and speech disorders: bulbar and pseudobulbar palsies.

13.3   Bulbar palsy: ipsilateral lower motor neuron lesion

This is caused by a lesion of the medulla (e.g. vascular, multiple sclerosis, motor neuron disease) which involves the nucleus ambiguus and the hypoglossal nucleus. There would be an ipsilateral lower motor neuron lesion of the muscles of the tongue and pharynx. Chewing, swallowing and speaking would be affected. Because the nuclei concerned are in the medulla or bulb, this is called a bulbar palsy.

13.4   Medullary syndromes

Lateral medullary syndrome (Wallenberg's or posterior inferior cerebellar artery syndrome)

This is caused by thrombosis of the posterior inferior cerebellar artery (PICA). Since this supplies the upper lateral medulla, some of the symptoms are explicable on the basis of the involvement of the spinal part of the trigeminal sensory nucleus and the nucleus ambiguus: disturbances of facial temperature sensation and bulbar palsy affecting speech and swallowing. There may also be cerebellar involvement and balance disorders (possible involvement of cochlear and vestibular nuclei). The lateral spinothalamic tract conveying pain and temperature sensation from the contralateral trunk and limbs may also be involved.

Medial medullary syndrome

This involves the hypoglossal nucleus, corticospinal tract and medial lemniscus. The medial medulla is supplied by the anterior spinal artery.

The lateral medullary syndrome is more likely to cause sensory symptoms, and the medial medullary syndrome more likely to cause motor syndromes: look again at Section 1.10 for the reasons for this.

13.5   Pseudobulbar palsy: contralateral upper motor neuron lesion

Interruption of the upper motor neuron pathways any-where between the cortex and the medulla (e.g. internal capsule, cerebral peduncles) will affect contralateral muscles of the tongue and pharynx. Since this presents as a disorder of the muscles of speech and swallowing, it is at first sight similar to a bulbar palsy, but being an upper motor neuron lesion, it is caused by a lesion on the opposite side. For these reasons it is known as a pseudobulbar palsy.

13.6   Broca's motor speech area

This is the area of motor cortex which controls the muscles of speech. It is immediately above the lateral fissure, deep to the pterion, usually in the dominant hemisphere (normally the left). Damage (e.g. occlusion of a branch of the middle cerebral artery) leads to motor speech aphasia (aphasia – wordless).

Chapter 14

THE GLOSSOPHARYNGEAL
NERVE (IX)

14.1   Functions

From a clinical point of view, the glossopharyngeal nerve is unimportant except for its role in the gag reflex. The main function of the glossopharyngeal nerve is the sensory supply of the oropharynx and posterior part of the tongue.

Its other functions are the motor supply to stylopharyngeus; conveying parasympathetic fibres part of the way to parotid gland and sensory supply from the carotid sinus, carotid body, and (sometimes) skin of the external acoustic meatus and tympanic membrane.

14.2   Origin, course and branches (Fig. 14.1)

- From medulla by a vertical series of rootlets lateral to olive, above and in series with those of X and XI.
- Passes through jugular foramen (middle portion). Two sensory ganglia: superior and petrosal (inferior).
- Parasympathetic axons from inferior salivatory nucleus to otic ganglion (for parotid gland) enter tympanic branch (see Chapter 17). May also convey sensory fibres from ear.
- Nerve descends in neck, supplying stylopharyngeus and carotid body.
- Passes between internal and external carotid arteries to enter pharynx. Sensory fibres to **pharyngeal plexus** supplying mucosa of pharynx and posterior tongue.

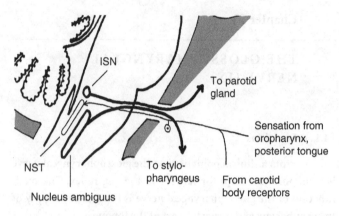

Fig. 14.1 Glossopharyngeal nerve.

Thick line: parasympathetic fibres from inferior salivatory nucleus
  (ISN) to otic ganglion for parotid gland, and branchiomotor fibres
  to stylopharyngeus.
Thin line: visceral sensory fibres passing to nucleus of solitary
  tract (NST).

14.3   The third branchial arch

The glossopharyngeal nerve is the nerve of the third
branchial arch which gives rise to the lower part of the hyoid bone
and the stylopharyngeus muscle. Arterial components of the third
arch form part of the common and internal carotid arteries thus
explaining the carotid sinus innervation.

14.4   Nerve fibres and nuclei

Visceral sensory fibres: to nucleus of the solitary tract.
Sensory fibres, including taste, from oropharynx, posterior tongue
and carotid body chemoreceptors. Cell bodies in petrosal ganglion.
Central processes pass to nucleus of the solitary tract.

Branchiomotor fibres: from nucleus ambiguus to stylopharyngeus.

Parasympathetic fibres: from inferior salivatory nucleus.
Preganglionic axons from inferior salivatory nucleus to auriculotemporal nerve and otic ganglion. Postganglionic fibres enter parotid gland. See Chapter 17.

Somatic sensory fibres: to nuclei of the trigeminal nerve.
From variable portion of skin in external ear, axons pass in tympanic branch to main trunk of IX. Cell bodies in superior ganglion of IX. Central processes pass to the sensory trigeminal nuclei.

14.5   Clinical notes and clinical testing

Gag reflex
Sensation supplied by the glossopharyngeal nerve is different in quality to that supplied by the trigeminal. Place a finger on the anterior part of the tongue (V) and then the posterior part (IX) to demonstrate this. The gag reflex is mediated by the glossopharyngeal (afferent limb) and the vagus (efferent limb). It is a functional test of both nerves.

Chapter 15

THE VAGUS NERVE (X)

15.1 Functions

The main functions of the vagus are phonation and swallowing. It also transmits cutaneous sensory fibres from the posterior part of the external auditory meatus and the tympanic membrane.

It supplies the gut tube as far as the splenic flexure of the transverse colon (roughly), and the heart, tracheobronchial tree and abdominal viscera. These fibres, though, are by no means essential to life, whatever others may tell you, since they can be cut, as in vagotomy. And do you suppose heart surgeons reconnect vagal branches during transplant operations? Of course not.

15.2 Origin, course and branches (Fig. 15.1)

The vagus is the most extensively distributed of all cranial nerves. Its name reflects both its wide distribution and the type of sensation it conveys (Latin: vagus – vague, indefinite, wandering).

- Arises from **medulla** by rootlets lateral to olive.
- Leaves posterior cranial fossa through jugular foramen (middle portion). In and below foramen are two sensory ganglia: jugular and nodose, containing cell bodies of sensory fibres. Auricular branch passes through canal in temporal bone and conveys sensory fibres from **external acoustic meatus and tympanic membrane**.

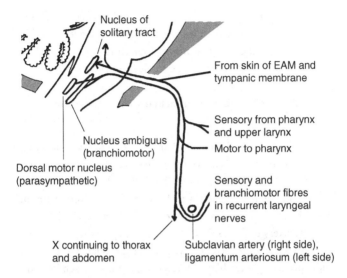

Nucleus of
solitary tract

From skin of EAM and
tympanic membrane

Sensory from pharynx
and upper larynx

Motor to pharynx

Nucleus ambiguus
(branchiomotor)

Dorsal motor nucleus
(parasympathetic)

Sensory and
branchiomotor fibres
in recurrent laryngeal
nerves

X continuing to thorax
and abdomen

Subclavian artery (right side),
ligamentum arteriosum (left side)

Fig. 15.1 Vagus nerve.

- Descends in **carotid sheath** posteriorly behind internal jugular vein and internal/common carotid arteries. Gives **pharyngeal branches**, and superior laryngeal nerve which has internal (sensory above vocal cords) and external (cricothyroid) branches.
- **Cardiac** (slowing heart rate) and tracheal (sensory) branches arise in the root of neck and upper thorax.
- **Recurrent laryngeal nerves** arise in superior mediastinum: left related to ligamentum arteriosum, right to subclavian artery. Both ascend between trachea and oesophagus to laryngeal muscles (not cricothyroid) and sensation of larynx below vocal cords, trachea, oesophagus.
- Forms **oesophageal plexus**. Enters abdomen through oesophageal hiatus in diaphragm as anterior and posterior trunks and

88 Glossopharyngeal, vagus and accessory nerves

contributes fibres to abdominal viscera and to coeliac, superior
mesenteric and myenteric plexuses. Branches pass in lesser omen-
tum alongside lesser curvature of stomach to innervate pyloric
antrum (**nerves of Latarjet**), and to give hepatic branches.

15.3 The fourth and sixth branchial arches: embryological considerations

The vagus is the nerve of the fourth and sixth branchial
arches. Structures derived from these include the pharyngeal and
laryngeal cartilages and muscles. The sixth arch artery on the left
gives rise to the ductus arteriosus (ligamentum after birth) around
which the left sixth arch nerve, the recurrent laryngeal, is caught
when the artery descends. The sixth arch artery on the right degen-
erates, so the right recurrent laryngeal nerve is related to the most
caudal persisting branchial arch artery, the fourth, which becomes
the right subclavian. The motor function of the vagus in the neck
is branchiomotor (special visceral motor): motor function in the
thorax and abdomen is parasympathetic (general visceral motor).

15.4 Nerve fibres and central connections

Branchiomotor fibres: from nucleus ambiguus
Nucleus ambiguus in medulla: branchiomotor nucleus of the third,
fourth and sixth branchial arches. Axons pass to muscles of pharynx
and larynx.
Parasympathetic fibres: from dorsal motor nucleus of vagus.
Dorsal motor nucleus of vagus (DMNX) in medulla gives preganglionic axons to innervate heart and thoracoabdominal viscera
(foregut and midgut). Cell bodies of postganglionic neurons are
generally in wall of destination organ, for example cardiac, myenteric plexuses.

Somatic sensory fibres: to sensory nuclei of the trigeminal nerve
From posterior wall of external auditory meatus and posterior portion of external surface of tympanic membrane, fibres pass in
auricular branch of X to main trunk in jugular foramen. Cell bodies in jugular (superior) ganglion. Central axonal processes pass to
trigeminal sensory nuclei.
Visceral sensory fibres: to nucleus of the solitary tract.
Taste fibres from epiglottic area, visceral sensory fibres from
hypopharynx, larynx, oesophagus, trachea, thoracoabdominal viscera and aortic baro- and chemo-receptors. Cell bodies in nodose
(inferior) ganglion. Central axonal processes pass to nucleus of
solitary tract.

15.5   An alternative view of the vagus

The vagus controls the entry into the gut tube (swallowing), and mediates sensation of most of the gut tube. This includes
the bronchial tree (a gut tube derivative). What about the heart?
This develops from heart tubes formed by angiogenetic cells initially
found in the wall of the yolk sac, from which the gut tube develops.
The yolk sac seems to be a common theme here. Perhaps we have
been too eager to over-analyze the vagus into parasympathetic,
branchiomotor, and so on. Perhaps the "big picture" is that the
vagus is the yolk sac nerve; the nerve of sustenance. Perhaps it is as
simple as that.

15.6   Clinical notes

1 *Gag reflex*
   See Section 14.5.

2 *Palatal elevation*

Observing the elevation of the palate when a subject says "ah" tests the motor function in the glossopharyngeal and vagus nerves.

3 *Vagal reflexes: coughing, vomiting, fainting*

Irritation of the skin on the posterior wall of the external auditory meatus (supplied by the vagus) can cause coughing (X: bronchial tree sensation), vomiting (X: alimentary canal sensation) or syncope (reflex bradycardia).

4 *Referred pain*

Pain from the pharynx and/or larynx may be referred to the ear. This is a characteristic presentation of hypopharyngeal tumours.

5 *Vocal cords*

Movements of the vocal cords are effected by the vagus. Laryngeal speech indicates that the vagus is intact at least to the level of the upper thorax. The mediastinal course of the left recurrent laryngeal nerve means that left mediastinal tumours may present as voice changes.

6 *Thyroid arteries*

The arteries of the thyroid gland are closely related to the laryngeal branches of the vagus. The superior laryngeal artery is related to the external laryngeal nerve near the origin of the artery, and the recurrent laryngeal nerve is related to the inferior thyroid artery close to the gland. This is relevant to thyroid surgery. Damage to the recurrent laryngeal nerves at this point nearly always affects fibres innervating the vocal cord abductors before those affecting adductors. This is serious, since if abduction is lost, the cords will be adducted and breathing will be difficult.

7 *Vagotomy*

Vagotomy was performed in patients with gastric ulcers to reduce gastric acid secretion by the stomach, and to decrease stomach emptying by preventing terminal antral contraction. Sometimes only the nerves of Latarjet were sectioned.

8 *Manipulation at surgery*

This may cause a reflex bradycardia.

15.7   Clinical testing

If speech is normal, the vagus nerves are fine. Tradition and convention, however, often demand the charade of testing them.

1 Listen to speech.
2 Gag reflex (see Section 14.5).
3 Testing palatal, pharyngeal movements, and listening to speech are tests of motor components of IX, X and cranial XI (see later). They are thus tests of the nucleus ambiguus.

Chapter 16

THE ACCESSORY NERVE (XI)

16.1 Parts and functions

The accessory nerve has two parts: cranial and spinal. Oddly enough, when clinicians refer to the eleventh cranial nerve, or accessory nerve, they almost always mean spinal accessory, which is not really a cranial nerve at all!

Cranial accessory

This arises from a caudal extension of the nucleus ambiguus by rootlets below and in series with those of IX and X. It joins the vagus, from which it is functionally indistinguishable (its name: accessory vagus). Some people hold that the muscles of the larynx and pharynx are innervated by the cranial accessory, leaving the vagus 'proper' with parasympathetic fibres only, but this is not certain. Clinically, such distinctions are unnecessary in any case, since when something goes wrong, it tends to affect a large area of the brain stem such that X and XI are likely to be affected along with other nerves. This book considers the cranial accessory no more.

Spinal accessory

Note: This is the one to remember.

This is motor to the muscles bounding the posterior triangle of the neck: **sternocleidomastoid and trapezius**.

16.2   Origin and course of spinal accessory (Fig. 16.1)

- Rootlets from **upper four or five segments of spinal cord** continue series of rootlets of IX, X and cranial XI.
- Emerge between ventral and dorsal spinal nerve roots, just behind denticulate ligament.
- **Ascends through foramen magnum** to enter posterior cranial fossa.
- Briefly runs with cranial XI before emerging through jugular foramen (middle compartment).
- Passes deep to sternocleidomastoid which it supplies.
- Enters roof of posterior triangle of neck. Surface marking in posterior triangle: one third of way *down* posterior border of sternocleidomastoid to one third of way *up* anterior border of trapezius.

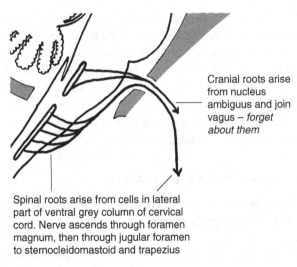

Cranial roots arise from nucleus ambiguus and join vagus – *forget about them*

Spinal roots arise from cells in lateral part of ventral grey column of cervical cord. Nerve ascends through foramen magnum, then through jugular foramen to sternocleidomastoid and trapezius

Fig. 16.1 Accessory nerve.

16.3   Nerve fibres and nuclei: what fibre types are present?

Cell bodies of spinal accessory motor neurons are in the lateral part of the ventral grey horn of the cervical cord in, apparently, a caudal extension of the nucleus ambiguus. Other muscles innervated by the nucleus ambiguus are classed as branchiomotor, yet not everyone is comfortable with this categorization for trapezius and sternocleidomastoid since it is not clear from which (if any) branchial arch they arise. It is intriguing to note, though, that branchial arch muscles are concerned with the cranial end of the gut tube and with nutrition, and the spinal accessory innervates muscles that move the head and neck when you are searching for food (e.g. consider a giraffe).

16.4   Clinical notes

The accessory nerve is vulnerable in the posterior triangle as it crosses the roof. Such injuries result in paralysis of trapezius (but not sternocleidomastoid which it has already supplied) and thus shoulder abduction beyond 90° involving scapular rotation is impaired (hair grooming, etc.). The accessory nerve may be damaged in dissection of the neck for malignant disease, in biopsy of enlarged lymph nodes in and around the posterior triangle, or in penetrating injuries to this region.

16.5   Clinical testing of spinal accessory

1 Ask the patient to shrug the shoulders (trapezius) against resistance.
2 Ask the patient to put hand on head (trapezius: shoulder abduction beyond 90°).
3 Ask the patient to move the chin towards one shoulder against resistance (contralateral sternocleidomastoid).

PART IV

AUTONOMIC COMPONENTS OF CRANIAL NERVES, TASTE AND SMELL

Chapter 17

PARASYMPATHETIC COMPONENTS AND TASTE SENSATION

17.1 Introduction

Except for the parasympathetic pathway to the eye, from a clinical point of view, these pathways are unimportant. However, they are intriguing, and understanding them might bring you satisfaction. But those to the eye are important (see Edinger–Westphal nucleus under Section 17.3).

Parasympathetic and taste pathways are considered together in this book because they share some peripheral pathways, particularly those that pass between branches of two different cranial nerves (e.g. chorda tympani, petrosal nerves). Also, on a more pedantic level, they are regarded as visceral functions – general visceral efferent (parasympathetic) and special visceral afferent (taste). Although the pathways are of great embryological interest, they matter very little clinically: as an example of this, deliberate section of the chorda tympani may have to be performed in ear surgery, and although food and drink may lose some savour, and the patient may subsequently suffer from a dry mouth, life continues much as before. This is a nuisance and may be inconvenient, but unless you are a *bon vivant* (to which we all may aspire) it is unlikely to be devastating.

17.2 Parasympathetic components (Table 17.1)

These innervate:
- the ciliary muscle and constrictor pupillae muscles;
- lacrimal and salivary glands;

Table 17.1. Parasympathetic components of cranial nerves.

Brain stem nucleus	Nerve of preganglionic fibres	Ganglion (synapses)	Nerve of post-ganglionic fibres	Functions
Edinger–Westphal (midbrain)	Oculomotor III	Ciliary	Nasociliary Va, short ciliary	Ciliary muscle: accommodation of lens, etc.; pupilloconstriction
Salivatory: superior (pons)	Facial VII, greater petrosal	Pterygopalatine	Zygomatic Vb, lacrimal Va	Secretomotor: lacrimal gland
			Nasal, palatine Vb	Secretomotor: nasal, palatine glands
	Facial VII, chorda tympani	Submandibular	Lingual Vc	Secretomotor: submandibular, sublingual glands
Salivatory: inferior (upper medulla)	Glossopharyngeal IX, lesser petrosal	Otic	Auriculotemporal Vc	Secretomotor: parotid gland
Dorsal motor nucleus of vagus (medulla)	Vagus X	Cardiac, myenteric	Very short, on or in target organs	Heart; foregut and midgut muscle and glands

- the sinuatrial node of the heart; and
- glands and muscles of the alimentary canal as far distally as the junction between midgut and hindgut (approximately the splenic flexure of the colon) (see Section 15.2).

We have already noted that parasympathetic fibres pass from branches of one cranial nerve to those of another and, for structures in the head, all postganglionic parasympathetic fibres, irrespective of their origin, attain their destinations in branches of the trigeminal nerve. These pathways are described below. Table 17.1 summarizes parasympathetic connections and ganglia.

17.3 Parasympathetic pathways in the head (Fig. 17.1)

1 Edinger–Westphal nucleus (III), ciliary ganglion, iris, ciliary body. This is important (see Chapter 22):
- Edinger–Westphal nucleus on rostral aspect of oculomotor nucleus in midbrain.
- Axons pass in oculomotor (III) nerve, inferior division, to ciliary ganglion (synapse).
- Postganglionic axons to iris and ciliary muscles in nasociliary and short ciliary nerves.
- Pupillary constriction (miosis), ciliary muscle contraction.

2 Superior salivatory nucleus (VII), greater petrosal nerve, pterygopalatine ganglion, lacrimal, nasal, palatine glands:
- Superior salivatory nucleus, cerebellopontine angle, internal auditory meatus (IAM), VII, greater petrosal nerve, carotid canal/foramen lacerum, greater petrosal nerve, pterygoid canal (with sympathetic fibres, deep petrosal nerve (see Section 19.2)).
- Pterygopalatine fossa, pterygopalatine ganglion (synapse).

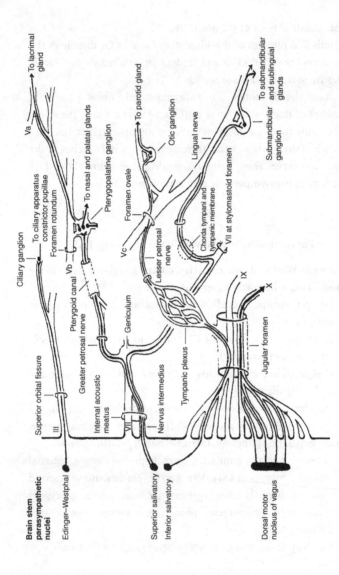

Fig. 17.1 Head and neck parasympathetics pathways. (Reprinted from Clinical Anatomy by Stanley Monkhouse, page 234 (2001) with permission from Elsevier.)

- Postganglionic fibres: (a) zygomatic nerve (Vb), inferior orbital fissure, lacrimal nerve (Va), lacrimal gland; (b) nasal, palatine branches (Vb) to nasal, palatine glands.

3 Superior salivatory nucleus (VII), chorda tympani, lingual nerve, submandibular ganglion, submandibular, sublingual glands:

- Superior salivatory nucleus, cerebellopontine angle, IAM, VII, facial canal, chorda tympani, crosses tympanic membrane on mucosal (medial) aspect, petrotympanic fissure, infratemporal fossa.
- Lingual nerve, submandibular ganglion (synapse).
- Postganglionic fibres to submandibular, sublingual glands.

4 Inferior salivatory nucleus (IX), lesser petrosal nerve, otic ganglion, auriculotemporal nerve, parotid gland:

- Inferior salivatory nucleus in upper medulla, glossopharyngeal (IX) nerve, jugular foramen, tympanic branch, tympanic plexus on medial wall of tympanic cavity, lesser petrosal nerve passes extradurally, through foramen ovale (or a hole of its own).
- Otic ganglion, auriculotemporal (Vc) nerve.
- Postganglionic fibres innervate parotid gland.

5 Dorsal motor nucleus of vagus (X), cardiac, pulmonary and myenteric (Meissner's, Auerbach's) ganglia, bronchial and cardiac muscle, smooth muscle of foregut and midgut.

These are not considered further in this text.

17.4   Taste fibres and pathways (Fig. 17.2)

Taste fibres enter the brain stem in VII, IX and X. Those entering through VII begin their journeys from taste buds in branches of Vb and Vc. They thus mirror some of the parasympathetic pathways described above, travelling from branches of one cranial nerve

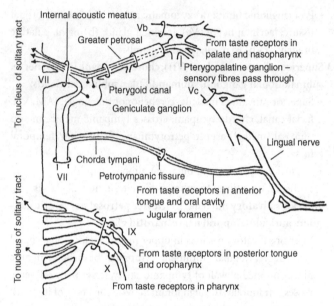

Fig. 17.2 Taste pathways. (Reprinted from Clinical Anatomy by
Stanley Monkhouse, page 235 (2001) with permission from
Elsevier.)

to another in nerves which also conduct parasympathetic fibres in
the opposite direction (e.g. chorda tympani, greater petrosal nerve).

Neurons conducting taste sensation centrally have cell bodies
in the sensory ganglia of the nerves through which they enter the
brain stem. Within the brain stem, as with all visceral sensation,
axons pass to the **nucleus of the solitary tract** (NTS).

1 In facial nerve (VII):
  • From anterior portion of tongue and neighbouring mucosa:
    – Taste buds in anterior portion of tongue and oral cavity.
    – Lingual nerve (Vc), chorda tympani, across tympanic mem-
      brane, VII in temporal bone, cell bodies in geniculate ganglion.

- Central processes through nervus intermedius, brain stem at cerebellopontine angle to NTS.

Compare this with parasympathetic fibres to submandibular ganglion (see Superior salivatory nucleus (VII) chorda tympani under Section 17.3).

- From the palate and nasopharynx:
  - Taste buds in palate, palatine branches of Vb.
  - Taste buds in nasopharynx, pharyngeal branches of Vb.
  - Fibres pass into pterygopalatine fossa, without interruption through pterygopalatine ganglion into pterygoid canal and greater petrosal nerve, VII in temporal bone, cell bodies in geniculate ganglion.
  - Central processes through nervus intermedius, brain stem at cerebellopontine angle to NTS.

Compare this course with that of parasympathetic fibres to pterygopalatine ganglion (see Superior salivatory nucleus (VII) greater petrosal nerve under Section 17.3).

2 In glossopharyngeal nerve (IX): from posterior tongue, oropharynx

- Taste buds in posterior part of tongue and oropharynx.
- IX, cell bodies in sensory ganglia of IX.
- Central processes to NTS.

3 In vagus nerve (X): from epiglottic region, hypopharyngeal wall

- Taste buds in epiglottic region and hypopharyngeal wall.
- X, cell bodies in sensory ganglia of X.
- Central processes to NTS.

17.5   Chorda tympani, branchial arches and petrosal nerves

The chorda tympani connects the facial and mandibular nerves, respectively the nerves of the second and first branchial arches. During embryonic development, each of the nerves of branchial arches 2, 3, 4 and 6 gives off a branch which pass into the territory of the preceding (cranial) branchial arch (second arch to first arch, third arch to second arch etc). Since, in order to take such a course, these branches pass from the caudal to the cranial sides of the slit between two adjacent branchial arches (Latin: *trema* means slit), these nerves are known as the pretrematic branches.

The chorda tympani is generally accepted as the pretrematic branch of the second branchial arch nerve. It passes from second arch tissue to first arch tissue through the tympanic membrane which is itself in the trema between the first and second arches. It contains two types of visceral fibre: afferent (taste) and efferent (parasympathetic). The embryological origin of the petrosal nerves is less certain.

17.6   Clinical notes

1 *Frey's syndrome*

   After parotidectomy, cut ends of postganglionic fibres begin to grow. Should these sprouting fibres find their way into Schwann cells sheaths occupied before surgery by sympathetic fibres, stimuli normally producing salivation will instead induce sweating over the site of the parotid. This is Frey's syndrome (gustatory sweating) (see Section 14.4).

2 *Runny eyes, streaming nose*

   Runny eyes, runny and blocked up nose might be produced by overactivity of the pterygopalatine ganglion. This is why the ganglion is sometimes called the *hay fever ganglion* although these symptoms are usually allergic.

17.7   Clinical testing of visceral components

1 *Salivary glands*

Ask the patient to suck something bitter (such as a lemon) to provoke salivary secretion. This is sometimes done to try to locate the position of a calculus in the duct of a salivary gland, usually the submandibular, but is not done to test the neural pathways since, as we have said, who cares?

2 *Taste*

Testing taste is possible but hardly worth the trouble.

Chapter 18

SMELL: THE OLFACTORY NERVE (I)

18.1 Introduction

The olfactory nerve transmits olfactory impulses from the olfactory epithelium of the nose to the brain. What is usually referred to as the olfactory nerve is properly the olfactory tract and bulb, and is an outgrowth of the forebrain. Primary sensory neurons are bipolar and are confined to the olfactory epithelium. Their central processes make up the numerous nerves which pass through the cribriform plate of the ethmoid bone. They synapse with secondary sensory neurons forming the olfactory bulb and tract. Olfaction is inextricably linked with taste; their central connections are poorly defined.

18.2 The olfactory nerves, bulb and tract (Fig. 18.1)

From olfactory epithelium in sphenoethmoidal recess and neighbouring area of nasal cavity, numerous **olfactory nerves** pass through cribriform plate and dura mater to: **olfactory bulb** situated over cribriform plate, which is site of origin of **olfactory tract** on inferior surface of frontal lobe, above orbital plate of frontal bone.

18.3 The olfactory pathway

• Smells stimulate peripheral processes of olfactory neurons.

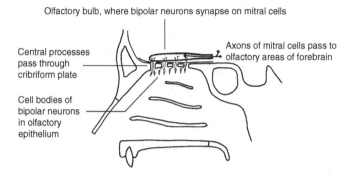

Olfactory bulb, where bipolar neurons synapse on mitral cells

Central processes pass through cribriform plate

Axons of mitral cells pass to olfactory areas of forebrain

Cell bodies of bipolar neurons in olfactory epithelium

Fig. 18.1 Olfactory pathways.

- Olfactory neurons are **bipolar** with cell bodies in olfactory epithelium.
- Central processes pass through cribriform plate and dura to …
- … synapse in olfactory bulb with secondary sensory neurons (mitral cells).

The olfactory bulb, tract, striae and connections

Axons pass posteriorly in olfactory tract, through olfactory striae to **limbic system** of brain, particularly the **uncus** and **amygdala** of the temporal lobe, thus providing connections with memory circuitry and much else.

18.4   Olfaction and taste

The pleasures of eating and drinking lie as much with smell as with taste: it is a common experience that an upper respiratory tract infection which interferes with the sense of smell impairs the enjoyment of food. Olfaction and taste are clearly closely linked and it is thought that from the nucleus of the solitary tract, to which taste fibres pass, axons project to the uncus to connect with olfactory centres.

18.5   Clinical notes

1 *Smells and the responses they can provoke*
  Evidence of olfactory connections to the limbic system are: (1) smells can trigger memories; (2) smells can provoke emotional responses; (3) smells have a role in sexual arousal.

2 *Anosmia*
  Head injuries which fracture the cribriform plate may tear olfactory nerves resulting in post-traumatic anosmia. Anosmia can also be caused by blockage of the nasal cavities, for example a nasal polyp or malignancy.

3 *Cerebrospinal fluid rhinorrhoea*
  Head injuries may tear the dura mater, leading to cerebrospinal fluid (CSF) leaking into the nasal cavity and dripping from the anterior nasal aperture. This should be considered if clear fluid issues from the nose after a head injury.

4 *Temporal lobe epilepsy*
  Diseases such as epilepsy in the areas to which the olfactory impulses project (e.g. the temporal lobe) may cause olfactory hallucinations. The smells which are experienced are usually unpleasant and are often accompanied by pseudo-purposeful movements associated with tasting such as licking the lips.

18.6   Clinical testing

Too much trouble – don't bother. You might just as well rely on the subjective opinion of the patient which is, after all, what matters most.

Chapter 19

THE SYMPATHETIC NERVOUS SYSTEM IN THE HEAD

Sympathetic fibres are not conveyed from the brain or brain stem in cranial nerves, but are found in distal branches of some cranial nerves. They are not usually considered components of cranial nerves, but they appear here for the sake of completeness.

19.1 Functions of the sympathetic system in the head

These are similar to those in the rest of the body: secretomotor to sweat glands, vasomotor (especially important for cerebral vessels), muscles of the hair follicles and so on. In addition, various structures in the eye receive a sympathetic innervation, particularly dilator pupillae and part of levator palpebrae superioris muscle.

19.2 Sympathetic pathways to cranial structures

Sympathetic nerve impulses leave the central nervous system only in the thoracolumbar region of the spinal cord. This means that if their destination is the head, they leave the spinal cord in upper thoracic spinal nerves and thence pass back up to the head. The sympathetic chain is the redistribution system by which means they ascend.

Preganglionic axons: T1, neck of first rib, cervical chain, synapse in superior cervical ganglion

- Preganglionic axons arise in lateral grey horn of T1 and/or T2 segments of spinal cord, and possibly also C8.

- Ventral roots of appropriate spinal nerves, spinal nerve, anterior primary ramus, white ramus communicans.
- Sympathetic chain at T1 ganglion near neck of first rib.
- Preganglionic axons for cranial structures do not synapse immediately, but ascend in sympathetic chain, posterior to carotid sheath, on surface or in substance of prevertebral muscles.
- Synapse in superior cervical ganglion (SCG) at rostral end of chain immediately below the base of skull.

Postganglionic axons
- From SCG, postganglionic fibres pass to wall of adjacent internal and external carotid arteries forming plexus around them.
- Plexus continues in walls of internal carotid, through carotid canal, into cranium and onto the walls of internal carotid artery and its branches.
- Postganglionic fibres delivered in walls of arteries to skin, eye, orbit, all cerebral arteries and other structures.

Cavernous sinus, orbital sympathetics, deep petrosal, on vertebral arteries
- As internal carotid artery passes through cavernous sinus, postganglionic fibres on its wall pass in fibrous strands which connect artery to lateral wall of sinus. Postganglionic fibres thus gain access to III, IV, Va, VI. This provides another route to orbit and eye and, through branches of ophthalmic nerve, to scalp.
- Orbital postganglionic fibres pass to levator palpebrae superioris muscle and to eyeball along III, Va, long and short ciliary nerves. Fibres traversing ciliary (parasympathetic) ganglion do so without synapsing.
- Deep petrosal nerve leaves carotid plexus in carotid canal. Joins greater petrosal nerve to form nerve of pterygoid canal to pterygopalatine fossa. Sympathetic fibres distributed in Vb to nose, pharynx, palate and face.

- Some fibres pass through cervical vertebral foramina transversaria with vertebral arteries to vessels of vertebrobasilar system.

19.3   Clinical notes

1 *Apical lung tumour: Horner's syndrome*

Any interruption of the sympathetic pathway to the eye would result in Horner's syndrome. Levator palpebrae superioris is partly supplied by the sympathetic system, and so would be weakened leading to drooping of the upper eyelid (ptosis). Sympathetic denervation of the iris would lead to unopposed pupillary constriction (miosis), and sympathetic denervation of sweat glands would result in an absence of sweating (anhidrosis). A tumour at the apex of the lung invading the neck of the first rib and interrupting the sympathetic chain would result in such signs. It may also damage T1 root of the brachial plexus causing weakness or paralysis of the small muscles of the hand with consequent impairment of grip.

2 *Cerebral vasculature and the sympathetic nervous system*

The regulation of cerebral blood flow is of great importance. Pathways described above regulate the calibre of all cerebral vasculature in response to physiological and other metabolic needs. This is performed by the sympathetic supply to arterial wall smooth muscle.

3 *Cervical sympathectomy*

This is interruption of the sympathetic pathways to the upper limb for peripheral vascular disease. The sympathetic chain is sectioned below T1 ganglion but the procedure is called cervical because it was often performed through a cervical incision. Providing that the chain is sectioned below T1 ganglion, which receives preganglionic impulses from the spinal cord, there will remain an adequate sympathetic supply to the head.

PART V

VISION, EYE MOVEMENTS, HEARING AND BALANCE: OPTIC, OCULOMOTOR, TROCHLEAR, ABDUCENS AND VESTIBULOCOCHLEAR NERVES

Chapter 20

THE OPTIC NERVE (II)

20.1 Sight

Sight is dependent not only on a substantial portion of the cerebral cortex, but also upon six cranial nerves (II–VII). Perception is the function of the retina, optic nerve, tract, radiation and cortex. The oculomotor, trochlear and abducens nerves move the eye. Eyeball sensations such as pain, touch and pressure are mediated by the ophthalmic nerve, and the facial nerve innervates orbicularis oculi muscle. This Chapter deals with the optic pathway: eye movements and their control come later.

20.2 The optic nerve

The optic pathway transmits visual impulses from the **retina to the brain**. The optic nerve is the name given to the pathway between the eyeball and the optic chiasma. It is an artificial subdivision of the optic pathway. Like the olfactory nerve (Chapter 18), the optic nerve is not really a nerve. It is an outgrowth of the diencephalon (the thalamic structures). As in the olfactory system, the primary sensory neurons are bipolar and are confined to the sensitive epithelium (retina), the axons of secondary sensory neurons forming the optic nerve, chiasma and tract.

20.3   Visual pathways (Fig. 20.1)

Described from the eyeball back to the forebrain attachment.

Retina

Two layers: neural (next to vitreous) and pigment (next to choroid).
Rods and cones in deepest parts of neural layer, with terminal
processes of rods and cones in contact with pigment layer. Rods and
cones synapse with bipolar cells (primary sensory neurons). Bipolar
cells, confined to retina, synapse on ganglion cells. Axons of ganglion
cells form optic nerve.

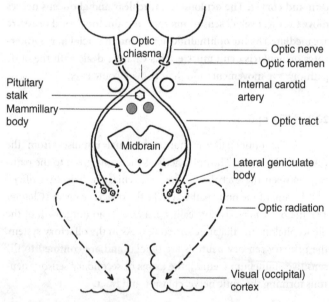

*Fibres to pretectal nuclei (see 20.4)
Fig. 20.1 Visual pathways.

Optic nerve, chiasma, tract

- **Optic nerve passes posteriorly from eyeball, surrounded by meninges, subarachnoid space, cerebrospinal fluid (CSF).** About half way between eyeball and optic canal, optic nerve is penetrated by central artery (branch of ophthalmic artery) and vein of retina.
- Optic nerve passes within common tendinous ring (giving origin to extrinsic ocular muscles) and leaves orbit through **optic canal** with ophthalmic artery below.
- Nerve surrounded by tube-like extension of three meningeal layers and subarachnoid space containing CSF.
- Optic nerves communicate at chiasma, anterior to hypophysis. At chiasma, fibres from nasal portion of each retina (impulses from temporal visual fields) cross to optic tract of opposite side.
- From chiasma, optic tracts extend back to lateral geniculate bodies (LGBs). Some axons bifurcate sending branches to midbrain for visual reflexes (see below).

LGB, optic radiation, visual cortex

- In LGB, axons of retinal ganglion cells synapse with cell bodies of neurons forming optic radiation.
- Axons pass backwards, skirting posterior limb of internal capsule and lentiform nucleus (thus retrolenticular).
- Axons pass around inferior horn of lateral ventricle and end in visual cortex (occipital lobe).

Consult a detailed neuroanatomy or neurophysiology text if you want more details.

20.4   Connections of visual pathway with midbrain

Some axons in the optic tracts bifurcate to give twigs which pass into the midbrain. These mediate visual reflexes and are connected to the pretectal nuclei (for the pupillary light reflex) and the superior colliculus and medial longitudinal fasciculus (for lens accommodation, eye movements, etc.). These reflexes and control mechanisms depend upon many other structures and are considered in Chapter 22.

20.5   Lesions of optic pathway

1 *Optic nerve*

   Section of one optic nerve causes blindness in one eye.

2 *Crossing fibres in chiasma*

   Destruction of crossing fibres in chiasma (e.g. pituitary tumour) causes blindness in the nasal retina of both eyes. This gives a bitemporal hemianopia (field loss).

3 *Pressure on lateral aspect of chiasma*

   Pressure on the lateral aspect of the chiasma (e.g. internal carotid aneurysm) affects fibres from the temporal retina of the ipsilateral eye, giving an ipsilateral nasal hemianopia. This is uncommon. Bilateral internal carotid artery aneurysms would cause a binasal hemianopia – even more uncommon.

4 *Optic tract or geniculate body*

   Destruction of the right optic tract or LGB would interrupt pathways from the temporal retina of the right eye and the nasal retina of the left eye. This would cause blindness in the left side of both visual fields. This is a homonymous hemianopia. Thus, destruction of the right optic tract would cause a left homonymous hemianopia.

5 *Optic radiation and visual cortex*

   Lesions of the optic radiation and visual cortex are more complex. *Consult a detailed neuroanatomy or ophthalmology text if you want more information.*

20.6   Other clinical notes

1 *Retinal signs of systemic disease*

The retina is the only part of the forebrain that can be viewed directly by an observer, so retinoscopy is an essential part of the neurological examination of a patient. Exudates, haemorrhages and abnormalities of blood vessels may be seen on retinoscopy and may be signs of generalized disease processes (e.g. diabetes, rheumatoid arthritis, etc.).

2 *Papilloedema and raised intracranial pressure*

Because the optic nerve in the orbit is surrounded by subarachnoid space containing CSF, raised intracranial pressure will compress the nerve. This will occlude the central vein before the central artery (venous blood is at a lower pressure). The retina will be engorged with blood and the optic disc will bulge into the vitreous. This is papilloedema, visible on retinoscopy – a reliable sign of raised intracranial pressure.

3 *Blood supply of visual cortex*

Although most of the visual cortex is supplied by the posterior cerebral artery, the cortical area which receives projections from the macula of the retina is generally supplied by both middle and posterior cerebral arteries. This is one of the explanations given for the phenomenon of macular sparing in which vision at the macula may be preserved even though the surrounding areas of the visual cortex are no longer functional.

4 *Retinal detachment*

The optic nerves and retina develop as a diencephalic outgrowth, the optic vesicle, which contains an extension of the diencephalic cavity, the third ventricle. As the two layers of the retina grow, they approach each other and the cavity is obliterated as the two layers become contiguous. The two layers give rise to the inner neural layer and the outer pigment layer. The potential space between them can open up in certain conditions, for example poor vascular perfusion. This is called retinal detachment; it causes blindness.

5 *Demyelinating diseases*

In the optic nerve, a brain outgrowth, myelin is produced by oligodendrocytes. The nerve may be affected in demyelinating diseases such as multiple sclerosis. This is not so for other cranial nerves in which myelin is manufactured by Schwann cells.

20.7   Clinical testing

Accurate assessments require the facilities of ophthalmology units, but crude assessment may be done by **confrontation**. This involves the examiner facing the patient, and both observing an object (usually the examiner's finger) held equidistant between patient and examiner. The object is at first held out of sight, and as it is brought towards the centre of the visual field from one extremity (right, left, top or bottom), the point at which it is first seen by both patient and examiner is noted. This method is based on comparing the patient's visual fields with those of the examiner, and thus assumes that the examiner is normal, at least in respect of his or her visual fields.

All crude tests of vision, of course, also depend on a normally functioning cornea, aqueous humour, iris, lens, vitreous humour, etc.

Chapter 21

THE OCULOMOTOR (III), TROCHLEAR (IV) AND ABDUCENS (VI) NERVES

The oculomotor (III), trochlear (IV) and abducens (VI) nerves innervate the extrinsic ocular muscles which move the eyeball. It is artificial to consider these nerves separately since both eyes move simultaneously to fix on a single point: eye movements are thus said to be **conjugate**. Furthermore, movement of the eyes to one side involves adduction of one eye and abduction of the other, demanding a sophisticated control mechanism (see Chapter 22).

21.1   Functions

These nerves innervate the extrinsic ocular muscles.

- *Oculomotor (III)*:
  - Superior division: levator palpebrae superioris (LPS), superior rectus.
  - Inferior division: medial rectus, inferior rectus, inferior oblique.
- *Trochlear (IV)*: superior oblique.
- *Abducens (VI)*: lateral rectus.

Through its parasympathetic components, the oculomotor nerve also causes **constriction of the pupil** (miosis) and has a role in **accommodation** of the lens (see Chapter 17).

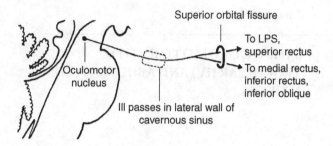

Fig. 21.1 Oculomotor nerve.

21.2   Origins and courses

All three nerves pass in the lateral wall of, or through, the cavernous sinus, and they enter the orbit through the superior orbital fissure.

Oculomotor nerve (III) (Fig. 21.1)

• From **interpeduncular fossa** of midbrain, passes through lateral wall of cavernous sinus. Superior and inferior divisions enter orbit through **superior orbital fissure** within common tendinous ring.

• Superior division supplies LPS, superior rectus (LPS is also partly innervated by sympathetic fibres – see Chapter 19).

• Inferior division supplies medial rectus, inferior rectus, inferior oblique. Also contains parasympathetic fibres from Edinger–Westphal nucleus to ciliary ganglion.

Trochlear nerve (IV) (Fig. 21.2)

• Smallest cranial nerve. From **dorsal aspect of midbrain** (uniquely), just below inferior colliculus. (Why? Did it once supply the pineal

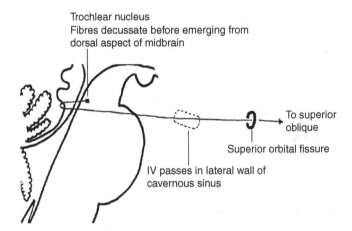

Trochlear nucleus
Fibres decussate before emerging from
dorsal aspect of midbrain

To superior
oblique

Superior orbital fissure

IV passes in lateral wall of
cavernous sinus

Fig. 21.2 Trochlear nerve.

gland – the so-called third eye, or perhaps first eye?) Passes around side of midbrain, through lateral wall of cavernous sinus, superior orbital fissure lateral to common tendinous ring.

• Passes above LPS to reach superior oblique.

Note: trochlear nerve is so called because superior oblique (which it supplies) is arranged as a pulley (Latin: *trochlea* – pulley).

Abducens nerve (VI) (Fig. 21.3)

• Arises from **pontomedullary junction** near midline, above rootlets of XII. Ascends to pass through cavernous sinus, on internal carotid artery, superior orbital fissure (within common tendinous ring).

• Supplies lateral rectus muscle.

Note: the abducens nerve is so called because lateral rectus abducts the eyeball.

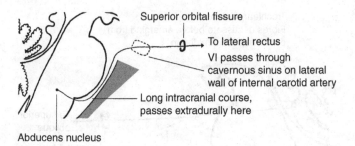

Superior orbital fissure

To lateral rectus

VI passes through
cavernous sinus on lateral
wall of internal carotid artery

Long intracranial course,
passes extradurally here

Abducens nucleus

Fig. 21.3 Abducens nerve.

21.3   Nerve fibres: nuclei

Somatic motor fibres – oculomotor, trochlear and abducens nuclei:
• Extrinsic ocular muscles are derived from pre-otic somites. Motor
  fibres innervating them, therefore, are somatic motor fibres and
  nuclei are somatic motor nuclei.
• Upper motor neuron input to nuclei of each side is bilateral.
• Nuclei also receive fibres from medial longitudinal fasciculus for
  control of eye movements, etc. (Chapter 22).
• Oculomotor nucleus: periaqueductal grey matter of midbrain,
  near midline, immediately ventral to aqueduct of Sylvius. Axons
  pass ventrally to emerge in the interpeduncular fossa.
• Trochlear nucleus in periaqueductal grey matter of midbrain,
  below oculomotor nuclei. Axons pass dorsally, decussating within
  midbrain dorsal to aqueduct.
• Abducens nucleus in pons, related to VII motor nucleus
  (Chapter 11).

Parasympathetic fibres in III: *Edinger–Westphal nucleus*
Edinger–Westphal nucleus on rostral margin of III nucleus. Receives
fibres from superior colliculi and pretectal nuclei (ocular reflexes,

Chapter 22). Preganglionic axons pass in III to ciliary ganglion (synapse). Postganglionic axons in short ciliary nerves to constrictor pupillae and ciliary muscles.

21.4   Clinical notes

1 *Visual reflexes and clinical testing* (see Chapter 22).
2 *Midbrain lesions: oculomotor nerve*
   Vascular or other lesions of the midbrain can affect the oculo-motor nerve. They may also affect the substantia nigra causing Parkinsonian symptoms (e.g. resting tremor), the red nucleus (also causing extrapyramidal symptoms), and the descending corticospinal fibres in the cerebral peduncles leading to a con-tralateral upper motor neuron lesions (UMNL). Benedikt's syn-drome involves the nerve as it passes through the red nucleus: oculomotor paralysis with contralateral extrapyramidal dyskine-sia. In Weber's syndrome the lesion is more ventral, also involving motor fibres in the cerebral peduncles: oculomotor paralysis is associated with contralateral UMNLs.
3 *Oculomotor nerve injury*
   The oculomotor nerve is liable to be stretched as it crosses the tentorial notch in cases of raised intracranial pressure. Complete section of the oculomotor nerve would lead to ptosis (partial paralysis of LPS), lateral squint (unopposed action of superior oblique and lateral rectus), pupillary dilatation (unopposed sympathetic activity), loss of accommodation and light reflexes. Irritation of the nerve may cause spasm of the muscles supplied by it (e.g. spasm of medial rectus leading to a medial squint).
4 *Oculomotor nerve injury: diabetes*
   It is not uncommon for diabetics to suffer from an acute vasculitis of the oculomotor nerve. This causes medial squint (somatic fibres) and ptosis (sympathetic fibres to LPS).

5 *Aneurysms of posterior cerebral artery: oculomotor nerve*

Just after the nerve leaves the midbrain it is intimately related to the posterior cerebral artery, aneurysms of which may compress the nerve leading to symptoms as described above.

6 *Trauma: trochlear nerve*

The trochlear nerve is the thinnest and most fragile nerve. It is vulnerable to trauma. Section of the nerve would result in the affected eye being turned medially.

7 *Intracranial disease: diagnostic usefulness of abducens nerve*

The abducens nerve, with a relatively low origin compared to its destination, has the longest intracranial course of any cranial nerve. It may be involved in fractures of the base of the skull or in intracranial disease. Section of the nerve would result in convergent squint (the eye abductor being paralyzed). See also *the effects of raised intracranial pressure: abducens nerve* below. Because of this long intracranial course it is often the first cranial nerve to be affected by intracranial disease. So, if you could only test one cranial nerve as part of a neurological investigation, this would be the one!

8 *Abducens and facial motor nuclei*

Diseases of the brain stem affecting the abducens nucleus may also involve fibres from the facial motor nucleus which loop around it.

9 *Gradenigo's syndrome: abducens nerve*

Since the abducens nerve passes over the apex of the petrous temporal bone, it may be affected by infections of the petrous temporal (petrositis), thus causing weakness of lateral rectus with consequent medial deviation of the ipsilateral eye (Gradenigo's syndrome: rare but interesting).

10 *The effects of raised intracranial pressure: oculomotor nerve*

When an expanding lesion above the tentorium causes raised intracranial pressure, the uncus of the temporal lobe may be squashed into the tentorial notch (herniation of the uncus). This compresses the midbrain which passes through the tentorial notch and the nearby oculomotor nerve. The result is pupillary dilatation (unopposed sympathetic action as the parasympathetic fibres in III are affected), at first unilateral and then bilateral. By this stage, the patient will already be unconscious.

11 *The effects of raised intracranial pressure: abducens nerve*
As intracranial pressure rises, the cerebrum may be forced backwards and downwards, thus stretching the nerve with its long intracranial course. A lateral rectus palsy (medial squint) would result. Because this may cause an erroneous diagnosis to be made, it is known as a false localizing sign.

12 *Cavernous sinus thrombosis: all three nerves*
Cavernous sinus thrombosis may occur as a result of an infection of any part of the head that drains through veins to the cavernous sinus (e.g. face, ear, etc.). It affects all the nerves that pass through or in the wall of the sinus (III, IV, Va, VI). The abducens nerve is usually affected first because it passes through the sinus, causing a paralysis of lateral rectus and a resultant medial squint. Involvement of the ophthalmic nerve may cause severe pain, and the condition may result ultimately in papilloedema and visual loss. Since the advent of antibiotic therapy, this condition is much less often encountered than formerly.

Chapter 22

VISUAL REFLEXES: THE CONTROL OF EYE MOVEMENTS; CLINICAL TESTING OF II, III, IV AND VI

22.1 Pupillary light reflex (Fig. 22.1, Table 22.1)

A light shone into either eye causes both pupils to constrict. This reflex is elicited on patients, conscious or unconscious, and it is, amongst other things, a crude test of brain stem function. Because of

Start at top left. Pass down left hand side, along bottom and up right hand side

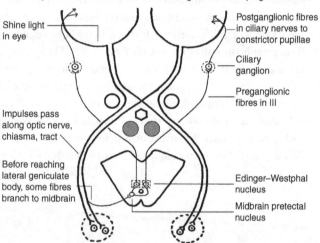

Shine light in eye

Postganglionic fibres in ciliary nerves to constrictor pupillae

Ciliary ganglion

Preganglionic fibres in III

Impulses pass along optic nerve, chiasma, tract

Before reaching lateral geniculate body, some fibres branch to midbrain

Edinger–Westphal nucleus

Midbrain pretectal nucleus

Fig. 22.1 Pupillary light reflex (study with Fig. 21.1). Start at top left, pass down left-hand side, along bottom and up right-hand side. (Reprinted from Clinical Anatomy by Stanley Monkhouse, page 269 (2001) with permission from Elsevier.)

Table 22.1. Pathways of light and accommodation reflexes.

Pupillary light reflex	Accommodation reflex
Retina	Retina
Optic nerve	Optic nerve
Optic chiasma	Optic chiasma
Optic tract, then branching fibres to: ↓	Optic tract, lateral geniculate body, optic radiation, visual cortex, association fibres to frontal lobes, fibres descend through anterior limb of internal capsule to:
Midbrain: pretectal nuclei	Midbrain: superior colliculus
Midbrain: Edinger–Westphal nucleus then ipsi- and contralateral to:	Midbrain: Edinger–Westphal nucleus then ipsi- and contralateral to:
Oculomotor nerve III	Oculomotor nerve III
Ciliary ganglion (synapse)	Ciliary ganglion (synapse)
Constrictor pupillae muscle for miosis	Muscles of iris and ciliary body

commissural connections, when light is shone into one eye, both pupils respond: the reflex is **consensual**. It does not involve the cortex; it may be performed on an unconscious subject. Only at the deepest levels of unconsciousness is there no response. Fixed dilated pupils are pupils which do not respond to light: they are a likely indicator of brain death. You need to know this pathway in some detail.

22.2   Accommodation reflex (Table 22.1)

In this reflex, focussing on an object near or far away results in changes of the size of the pupil (near: constricted; far: dilated) and the lens (near: more convex; far: less convex). These changes are equivalent to those made by photographers in stop adjustment and lens extension on a camera. You will realize that in the accommodation reflex perception is involved, unlike the pupillary light reflex, and thus the cortex is involved. There is also a degree of voluntary control since you can decide to focus on an object. The precise pathways are not fully understood, but those given in Table 22.1 are probable.

22.3 Argyll Robertson pupil

The Argyll Robertson pupil is one that accommodates but does not react to light. A comparison of the pathways for the accommodation reflex, which functions normally, and the pupillary light reflex, which does not, indicates that the lesion could be in: (a) the fibres that pass from the optic tract to the midbrain, (b) the pretectal nuclei or (c) that part of the Edinger–Westphal nucleus which deals with fibres from the pretectal nuclei.

22.4 Conjugate eye movements and their control

Eye movements involve nuclei of III, IV and VI integrated by mechanisms which include the frontal eye fields, the superior colliculus, the pontine gaze centre, the cerebellum, and the medial longitudinal fasciculus (MLF).

The **frontal eye fields** mediate voluntary eye movements and are responsible for saccadic movements by which means we search the visual fields for an object on which to fix. Saccades are so rapid that individual visual images are imperceptible until fixation has ensued. Frontal eye field stimulation causes conjugate movement of the eyes to the opposite side.

The **superior colliculi** on the dorsal aspect of the midbrain are involved in visual reflexes. This part of the brain stem is known as the tectum (Latin: roof): tectospinal and spinotectal tracts pass to and from the spinal cord.

The **MLF** extends from midbrain to cervical spinal cord. It integrates the nuclei of III, IV and VI with:

- ventral horn cells (motor) of the cervical spinal cord for the control of head and neck movements involved in visual fixation movements;
- vestibular nuclei (see Chapter 23);
- auditory nuclei (see Chapter 23);
- the cerebellum.

Consider what happens when you watch a fixed object from a moving vehicle. As the head and neck turn sideways, the **vestibular–ocular reflex** keeps your eyes fixed on the object. Impulses from the vestibular apparatus, and from the neck muscles by way of the spinal cord, pass to the MLF and the nuclei of III, IV and VI causing the extrinsic ocular muscles to bring about a series of **saccades** which, although imperceptible to you, continually reset the eyes on target. These connections are also brought into play in other circumstances: disorders of the vestibular apparatus (e.g. Ménière's disease – see Section 23.5), a loud noise, or pain mediated by a spinal nerve, can all result in reflex eye movements.

Nystagmus

The MLF is also connected to the cerebellum, and so can be affected in cerebellar disease producing abnormal eye movements. Disorders of any part of this system may lead to jerky eye movements – nystagmus. This can be regarded as ataxia of the eye muscles.

22.5   Internuclear ophthalmoplegia

This occurs when the MLF in the brain stem is damaged (e.g. multiple sclerosis). The nuclei of III, IV and VI become disconnected, and uncoordinated movements of the eyes result in strabismus (squints).

22.6   Clinical testing of eyes and eye movements

1 Pupillary light reflex. Shine a light into one eye and observe both pupils. This tests II, midbrain, III.
2 Corneal reflex tests Va, brain stem and VII.
3 Observe pupillary size: both should be equal. If not, there may be a lesion of III or midbrain.
4 Look for nystagmus. Nystagmus present on straight forward gaze is definitely abnormal. Nystagmus evident at the extremes of eye movements is only possibly abnormal.
5 Look for a squint. A lesion of the main trunk of the oculomotor, trochlear or abducens nerves will be obvious.
6 With the head stationary, the patient should be asked to follow with both eyes together an object moving not-too-quickly (e.g. the examiner's finger or a pen) as it describes a large square with both diagonals. Should any abnormality be observed, each eye may be tested more carefully. Or, if you want the easy way out, send the patient to an optician or ophthalmologist.

Chapter 23

THE VESTIBULOCOCHLEAR NERVE (VIII) AND AUDITORY AND VESTIBULAR PATHWAYS

23.1   Functions

Hearing and balance. The vestibulocochlear nerve is the sensory nerve for hearing (cochlear) and equilibration (vestibular). It is also known as the statoacoustic nerve.

23.2   Origin and course

Arises laterally in **cerebellopontine angle**. Passes with VII into **internal acoustic meatus** (temporal bone). Cochlear portion (anteriorly) and vestibular portion (posteriorly). Vestibulocochlear nerve does not emerge externally.

23.3   Cochlear nerve, auditory pathways and reflexes (Fig. 23.1)

Cochlear nerve and ganglion

- **Bipolar** primary sensory neurons (like olfactory and visual systems) originate from organ of Corti in basilar membrane in floor of cochlear duct (scala media).
- Cell bodies in **cochlear ganglion** situated in modiolus, or axis around which cochlea twists. Ganglion thus also known as spiral ganglion.
- Central processes pass in cochlear nerve to **cochlear nuclei**.

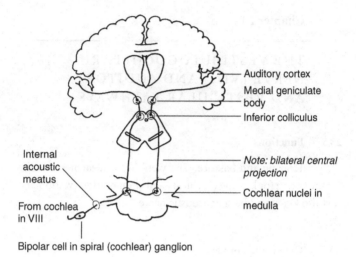

Fig. 23.1 Auditory pathways.

Cochlear nuclei – medial geniculate body – auditory cortex
- Cochlear nuclei laterally in floor of fourth ventricle.
- Subsequent sensory neurons pass **bilaterally** to **inferior colliculi** (tectum of midbrain) and **medial geniculate bodies** (diencephalon).
- Inferior colliculi concerned with auditory reflexes.
- Some neurons pass to other centres (e.g. medial longitudinal fasciculus, reticular formation, spinal cord) for integration with other systems.
- Ascending pathways are multisynaptic, other components being superior olive, trapezoid body, lateral lemniscus. Commissural fibres also occur between inferior colliculi, medial geniculate bodies.

- Axons from medial geniculate bodies project through internal capsule to **auditory cortex in upper part of temporal lobe** on inferior operculum, just below lateral fissure (territory of middle cerebral artery).

Note: visual system: lateral geniculate bodies, superior colliculi; auditory system: medial geniculate bodies, inferior colliculi.

Examples of auditory reflexes: when a loud noise is heard

- Extrinsic ocular muscles turn eyes towards source of sound – connections from inferior colliculi to superior colliculi, to the nuclei of oculomotor, trochlear and abducens nerves (in medial longitudinal fasciculus, etc.).
- Sudden inspiration and/or exclamation (startle reflex) – connections to spinal cord (tectospinal) and nucleus ambiguus (tectobulbar).
- Tensing of tympanic membrane and stabilization of the stapes, which directly impinges on cochlea – connections to trigeminal motor nucleus (tensor tympani) and facial motor nucleus (stapedius).
- May lead to arousal from sleep – connections to reticular formation.

23.4   Vestibular nerve, pathways and reflexes (Fig. 23.2)

The vestibular pathways are intimately connected with the cerebellum. These are some of the oldest neural pathways in the animal kingdom.

Vestibular nerve and ganglion: cerebellum

- **Bipolar** primary sensory neurons originate from hair cells in vestibular apparatus: saccule, utricle, semicircular ducts. Cell bodies in vestibular ganglion in temporal bone.

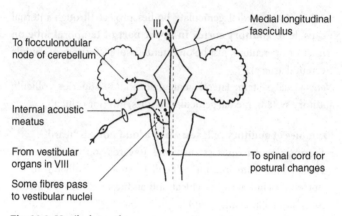

Fig. 23.2 Vestibular pathways.

- Central processes pass in vestibular nerve either directly to **cerebellum**, or to **vestibular nuclei** in medulla.
- Vestibular impulses pass to floccule, nodule, uvula, fastigial nucleus – the vestibulocerebellum, phylogenetically the oldest part of cerebellum.

Vestibular nuclei and connections
- Vestibular nuclei in floor of fourth ventricle.
- Fibres descend in vestibulospinal tracts to spinal cord, others pass to medial longitudinal fasciculus for integration with eye muscle nuclei.
- Other fibres from nuclei pass to cerebellum (in addition to those passing directly from vestibulocochlear nerve to cerebellum).
- Vestibular system projects to ventral posterior nucleus of thalamus and since we have a conscious awareness of stability in space, impulses may pass to parts of cerebral cortex.

Examples of vestibular reflexes
- Muscles act to counter unwanted movement – vestibulospinal connections.
- As we move progressively in one direction, slow eye movements in opposite direction are followed by rapid movements in same direction (for eyes to catch up). This is **nystagmus**. Connections to the nuclei of oculomotor, trochlear and abducens nerves (in medial longitudinal fasciculus).
- Connections also from vestibular pathways and cerebellum to **reticular formation** (arousal if necessary) including **vomiting centre** in medulla.

23.5   Clinical notes

Remember that within the inner ear, the cochlear duct is continuous with the saccule, utricle and semicircular ducts: they form an enclosed endolymph containing system derived from the otocyst. Cochlear disorders, therefore, may affect the vestibular system, and vice versa as follows:

1 *Conductive deafness*

This is deafness resulting from defective transmission of sound waves to the endolymph. It may be caused by blockage of the external acoustic meatus, a large perforation in the tympanic membrane (reducing its ability to pick up sound waves), impairment of ossicular movement (e.g. fluid in the tympanic cavity, ossicular joint disease, dislocation of the ossicular chain) or fixation of footplate of the stapes.

2 *Sensorineural deafness*

This is deafness resulting from disease of the cochlea, the vestibulocochlear nerve or the auditory pathway. It is clinically distinguishable from conductive deafness. It includes the deafness of old age (presbyacusis).

3 *Nerve deafness*

This is sensorineural deafness resulting specifically from disease of the vestibulocochlear nerve or the auditory pathways. If the auditory pathways are involved, the deafness is rarely profound because of the bilateral connections of the cochlear nuclei.

4 *Acoustic neuroma*

This is a tumour of Schwann cells on the vestibular nerve in the cerebellopontine angle. If the tumour grows in the internal acoustic meatus, it will compress both vestibulocochlear and facial nerves causing a nerve deafness and, eventually, an ipsi-lateral facial palsy.

5 *Stapedius paralysis: hyperacusis*

This leads to a peculiar echoing sensation even though sounds may not be particularly loud (hyperacusis) and it arises in facial nerve lesions; it may be the first symptom of disease (see Stapedius: hyperacusis under Section 11.7).

6 *Inability to localize sounds in space*

A unilateral lesion of the auditory cortex, though not resulting in profound deafness (because of bilateral pathways), may lead to difficulty in localizing the source of a sound. This is socially awkward and can be dangerous.

7 *Labyrinthine artery*

This is a branch of the vertebrobasilar system and enters the internal acoustic meatus to supply VII, VIII and the inner ear. Lesions of this artery, or of the vertebrobasilar system, can cause vertigo and unsteadiness. Narrowing of the vertebral arteries by either atherosclerosis or by cervical vertebral osteophytes may lead to these symptoms with neck movements.

8 *Nystagmus*

Disorders of the vestibular system, the cerebellum, and/or the medial longitudinal fasciculus in the brain stem, may lead to pathological nystagmus with slow eye movements in one direction followed by quick movements in the other. It requires investigation.

9 *Travel sickness*

This common condition illustrates the connections from the vestibular pathways and cerebellum to the vomiting centre in the medulla.

10 *Ménière's disease*

Prosper Ménière described a condition consisting of attacks of deafness, vertigo and tinnitus (noises in the head). It arises from an endolymph disorder and its symptoms reflect the endolymphatic continuity between cochlea, saccule, utricle and semicircular ducts.

23.6   Clinical testing

1 Simple tuning fork tests and audiometry distinguish between external and middle ear deafness (conductive) and inner ear and nerve deafness (sensorineural). The former usually is treatable, the latter usually is not.

2 Vestibular function can be tested by:

(a) electrical neurophysiological testing.

(b) a long established and still performed test, the caloric test, which involves irrigating the external auditory meatus with warm and cold water. Convection currents affect the lateral semicircular duct which provokes nystagmus. The duration of this can be measured and compared with results from a normal subject.

The best and easiest way to test the function of the vestibulocochlear nerve is to send the patient to the ENT clinic with, of course, a polite request.

FURTHER READING

You may wish to consult reference books for details on topics that interest you. There are so many books available that this list is only a lucky dip, others would choose differently.

For topographical anatomy: any large textbook, for example
Standring S et al. *Gray's Anatomy*. Churchill Livingstone, 2004. ISBN 0443071683.

For anatomical anomalies:
Hollinshead WH. *Anatomy for Surgeons. Vol. 1: The Head and Neck*, 3rd edition. Harper and Row, 1982.
Schäfer EA, Symington J, Bryce TH. *Quain's Elements of Anatomy*, Vol. III, 11th edition. Longmans, Green and Co, 1909.

For developmental anatomy:
Gilbert SF. *Developmental Biology*. Sinauer Associates, 2003. ISBN 0878932585.
Hamilton WJ, Boyd JD, Mossman HW. *Human Embryology*. The Macmillan Press Ltd, 1975.

For detailed neuroanatomy:
Kandel ER, Schwartz JH, Jessell TM. *Principles of Neural Science*. McGraw-Hill/Appleton & Lange, 2000. ISBN 0838577016.

Ranson SW, Clark SL. *Anatomy of the Nervous System*, 10th edition. WB Saunders and Company, 1959.

Butler AB, Hodos W. *Comparative Vertebrate Neuroanatomy: Evolution and Adaptation*. Wiley-Liss, 1996. ISBN 0471888893.

For clinical neurology:

Donaghy M (ed.). *Brain's Diseases of the Nervous System*. Oxford University Press, 2001. ISBN 0192626183.

INDEX

Entries are listed by terms in common use, thus trigeminal ganglion, not ganglion, trigeminal.

Printed in the United States
By Bookmasters